Pelvic Yoga:

An Integrated Program of Pelvic Floor Exercise
to Overcome Incontinence
and Support Overall Pelvic Floor Health

Also by Kimberlee Bethany Bonura, PhD, RYT:

From The Great Courses (www.thegreatcourses.com):

How to Stay Fit as You Age, with Kimberlee Bethany Bonura, PhD (2013).

DVDs / Video Downloads from Yoga by Kimberlee Bethany Bonura (www.drkimberleebonura.com):

Pelvic Yoga Basics, with Kimberlee Bethany Bonura (2012)

Power Pelvic Yoga, with Kimberlee Bethany Bonura (2012)

Pelvic Yoga on the Chair: Totally Chair Yoga, with Kimberlee Bethany Bonura (2012)

Pelvic Yoga for Pregnancy, with Kimberlee Bethany Bonura (2012)

Pelvic Yoga, with Kimberlee Bethany Bonura (2006 / 2010)

Pelvic Yoga on the Chair, with Kimberlee Bethany Bonura (2006 / 2010)

Chair Yoga, with Kimberlee Bethany Bonura (2006 / 2010)

Totally Chair Yoga, with Kimberlee Bethany Bonura (2006 / 2010)

CDs/ MP3s from Yoga by Kimberlee Bethany Bonura (www.drkimberleebonura.com):

Pelvic Yoga: Introduction to Pelvic Floor Exercise with a Yoga Floor Routine (2002 / 2010)

Chair Yoga with Standing Poses (2002 / 2010)

Textbooks:

Bonura, K.B. (2009). Yoga for Older Adults. Saarbrücken, Germany: VDM Verlag Publications.

Bonura, K.B. (2009). Academic Learning and Play. In R.P. Carlisle (Ed.), *Encyclopedia of Play*, Thousand Oaks, CA: Sage Publications.

Bonura, K.B. (2009). Memory and Play. In R.P. Carlisle (Ed.), *Encyclopedia of Play*, Thousand Oaks, CA: Sage Publications.

Green, L.B., & **Bonura, K.B**. (2007). The use of imagery in the rehabilitation of injured athletes. In D. Pargman (Ed.), *Psychological Bases of Sport Injuries*, 3rd Ed. Morgantown, WV: Fitness Information Technology.

Pelvic Yoga:

An Integrated Program of Pelvic Floor Exercise to Overcome Incontinence and Support Overall Pelvic Floor Health
2nd Edition

KIMBERLEE BETHANY BONURA, PhD, RYT

Yoga by Kimberlee Bethany Bonura

www.drkimberleebonura.com

info@drkimberleebonura.com

Copyright © 2002, 2012 Kimberlee Bethany Bonura

Copyright © 2nd Edition, 2013 Kimberlee Bethany Bonura

All rights reserved.

Pelvic Yoga is a trademark of Yoga by Kimberlee Bethany Bonura, LLC.

ISBN: **1481158368**
ISBN-13: **978-1481158367**

Without limiting the rights under copyright reserved above, no part of this publication may be reproduced, stored in, or introduced into a retrieval system, or transmitted, in any form, or by any means (electronic, mechanical, photocopying, recording, or otherwise) without the prior written permission of the copyright owner. The scanning, uploading, and distribution of this book via the Internet or via any other means without the permission of the copyright owner is illegal and punishable by law.

FOR KYRA AND ERIK

CONTENTS

Overview 1
Introduction to Pelvic Floor Exercise 2
   Anatomy and Physiology of the Pelvic Floor 2
   Pelvic Floor Exercises: Basics 3
      Pelvic Floor Exercises for Women 4
      Pelvic Floor Exercises for Men 6
   Three Techniques to Recognize Your Pelvic Muscles: 7
      (1)   Stop Test 7
      (2)   Finger Test 8
      (3)   Medical Exam 8
   Pelvic Floor Exercise Tips 9
   Mistakes to Avoid 11
   Four Advanced Pelvic Floor Exercise Techniques 12
      (1)   Contract-Release 12
      (2)   Quick-Flicks 12
      (3)   Long Holds 13
      (4)   Elevators 13
Pelvic Yoga—an Integrated Program of Pelvic Floor Exercise 16
   Yoga Breath 16
   Yoga Vision 17
   Pelvic Floor Exercise and Yoga Bandhas ("Locks") 18
      Ashtanga Yoga Root Lock 18
      Kundalini Energy 19
      Root Lock 19
      Sat Kriya 21
      Root Lock During Menstruation 23
      Stomach Lock 23
   Beginning Poses 24
      (1)   Simple Sitting Contract-Releases 24

	(2)	Cat-Cow Pose Contract-Release	26
	(3)	Child's Pose Quick-Flicks	28
	(4)	Chair Quick-Flicks	29
	(5)	Staff Pose with Long Holds	31
	(6)	Wind-Relieving Pose with Long Holds	32
	(7)	Mountain Pose Balance with Elevators	34
	(8)	Corpse Pose Elevator	36
Moderate Poses			38
	(1)	Perfect Posture Contract-Release (Tailor Pose)	38
	(2)	Camel Contract-Release	39
	(3)	Frog Pose Quick-Flicks	42
	(4)	Squatting, Legs Together, Quick-Flicks	44
	(5)	Squatting, Legs Apart, Elevator	45
	(6)	Cobbler's Pose Elevators	47
	(7)	Tree Pose Balance with Long Holds	48
	(8)	Bridge Pose with Long Holds	50
Advanced Poses			52
	(1)	Wide-Leg Sitting Forward Bend	53
	(2)	Happy Baby Pose	55
	(3)	Downward Facing Dog Pose	57
	(4)	Fish Pose	59
	(5)	Backbend (Wheel)	61
Supportive Yoga Exercises			64
Supportive Exercises for Abdominal Strengthening			64
	(1)	Stomach Contractions / Abdominal Lift	64
	(2)	Kundalini Sitting Twists	67
	(3)	Angle Balance and Wide-Leg Angle Balance	68
	(4)	Pelvic Yoga Bicycle	70
	(5)	Reclined Cobbler's Pose Crunches	71
	(6)	Boat Pose	73
	(7)	Airplane	76
	(8)	Locust	77

Supportive Exercises for the Thighs, Pelvis, and Buttocks 78
- (1) Warrior One 78
- (2) Crescent Pose 81
- (3) Warrior Two 82
- (4) Side-Angle Pose 84
- (5) Triangle 85
- (6) Eagle 87
- (7) Partial Pigeon 89
- (8) Sleeping Big-Toe Cycle 91

Supportive Exercise for the Back 94
- (1) Standing Spinal Rolls 94
- (2) Cow-Face Pose 95
- (3) Seated Spinal Twist 97
- (4) Cobra 99
- (5) Bow 100
- (6) Chinese Ancestor Worship 102
- (7) Reclining Twist (Knees Bent) 103
- (8) Supported Backbend 105

Yoga Walking Pelvic Floor Exercise 106

Pelvic Floor Meditation 109
- (1) Beginner: Spread Legs up the Wall Pose 110
- (2) Moderate & Advanced: Reclined Cobbler's Pose 113

Pelvic Yoga Quick Guide: Using Yoga for Pelvic Health 116

References 117

Suggested Internet Resources 122

Index 123

About the Author 125

KIMBERLEE BETHANY BONURA

ACKNOWLEDGMENTS

I would like to express my gratitude and appreciation to:

My mother, Sandra Hoirup Bethany.

My husband, Michael Bonura.

The yoga instructors and academic professors who have provided training, guidance, and mentorship in their areas of expertise.

The yoga students who have taken my classes and allowed me to share in their journey.

KIMBERLEE BETHANY BONURA

Note to the Reader

Please note the following important precautions before using this product.

Every effort has been made to ensure that the information in this book is complete and accurate. However, neither the publisher nor the author is engaged in rendering professional advice or services to the individual reader. The ideas, procedures, and suggestions in this book are not intended as a substitute for consulting with your physician. All matters regarding your health require medical supervision.

The material provided is intended as helpful information for preventative bladder and pelvic health. It is not intended to diagnose or treat any medical condition. Medical conditions should be discussed with a doctor, and pelvic/urinary issues should be discussed with an appropriate medical specialist.

Not all exercises are suitable for everyone, and this or any exercise program may result in injury. Consult with your physician before beginning this or any other exercise program. To reduce the risk of injury, never force or strain yourself during exercise. If you experience pain or discomfort during exercise, stop immediately and consult your physician.

Certain precautions apply to this or any other exercise program. Pregnant women should not practice twists, backbends, or breath-holding poses. Pregnant women should not lie flat on their backs in the second or third trimester. Pregnant women should consult with their obstetricians prior to beginning any exercise program.

Other precautions may apply to individuals with specific health issues. If you have any other chronic health condition(s), consult with your physician prior to beginning this, or any other, exercise program.

This program is sold without warranties or guarantees of any kind. Any liability, loss, or damage in connection with any use of this program, including but not limited to any liability, loss, or damage resulting from the information or suggestions in this book, or performance of the exercises described here, or the advice and information given here, is expressly disclaimed.

KIMBERLEE BETHANY BONURA

Foreword

Statistically, 10 to 15 percent of children eight to sixteen years old have nighttime wetting problems. Twenty-five percent of adults twenty-five to fifty-five years old have experienced leakage problems. Thirty-five to 40 percent of adults over sixty-five years old have leaking problems, and in nursing homes, over 50 percent are incontinent.

There are ways to prevent, control, and/or slow this process—with exercises, dietary changes, and good bladder habits. In cases where there is no structural defect, most individuals will improve with pelvic floor rehabilitation. Proper pelvic floor exercises include the contraction of the entire pelvic floor muscles, felt by squeezing the rectum and vagina simultaneously, with the frequency and types of exercises as prescribed by the practitioner. The muscles of the pelvic floor are no different from any other muscle; they need daily exercise to stay in shape and perform functionally. This program is just as beneficial for men as for women. The musculature is the same; the plumbing is a little different!

My best wishes to the readers and participants in this combined program of pelvic floor rehabilitation and yoga. Kudos to Kimberlee for combining a most valuable adjunct to yoga, and a gift to all women and men.

Kathleen A. Roth, PT, DPT
Owner, Tier 1 Physical Therapy and Sports Medicine
http://tier1pt.com/
El Paso, Texas

KIMBERLEE BETHANY BONURA

Overview

Pelvic Yoga facilitates optimum health of the urinary and reproductive systems by strengthening the pelvic floor. The focus is on preventing urinary incontinence, enhancing sexuality, and maintaining pelvic health. Men and women of all ages will benefit from a preventative program of pelvic exercises. For women who are pre- and post-pregnancy or pre- and post-menopause, the program is essential to overcome natural weakening of the pelvic floor caused by weight gain, stretching of pelvic muscles during pregnancy and delivery, and/or hormonal changes. Because male incontinence does occur, men will also benefit from Pelvic Yoga.

The program integrates pelvic floor exercises into a yoga practice designed to strengthen, tone, and increase flexibility in the muscles of the pelvis, abdomen, lower back, hips, and thighs. Pelvic floor exercises are a vital component of any health program and are particularly important to support reproductive and sexual well-being.

Additional practices, such as appropriate dietary choice, vitamin and herbal supplements, and bladder retraining activities, can also yield improvements in pelvic floor health. The suggested list of Internet resources at the end of this text provides credible sources of information to learn more about urinary incontinence, additional treatment options, and supportive activities.

Introduction to Pelvic Floor Exercise

Anatomy and Physiology of the Pelvic Floor

The pelvic floor is a "hammock" of several muscles, connected down the midline, extending from the base of the spine to the base of the pubic bone. The pubococcygeus muscles run from the tailbone to the pubic bone and help stop the flow of urine, suppress gas, and permit women to tighten the vagina. Interconnected muscles work together as a unit, with some muscles working strongly over long periods and other muscles only capable of working for short bursts. The pelvic floor supports the abdominal and pelvic organs, bladder, bowel, and uterus. Weakness in the pelvic muscles can be caused by weight gain; by accident or injury to the pelvic region; by hormonal changes, such as in pregnancy or menopause; and by pregnancy-induced weight gain. When the pelvic muscles slacken, pressure increases on the bladder, and the ability to hold the sphincter of the urethra declines, potentially causing urine leakage under pressure (sneezing, jumping, laughing, exercising, etc.). Loose pelvic muscles also indicate a stretched vaginal cavity, which lessens sexual pleasure during intercourse. However, the muscles of the pelvic floor are part of the voluntary nervous system, which means we have control over them and the ability to strengthen and build them.

In men, the bulbospongiosus surrounds the lower shaft of the penis, with the external sphincter ani curving back around the anus, and the two circular muscles connected at the center point of the perineal body. Because of the design of the male anatomy, men have a built-in protection against problems with incontinence. The prostate gland surrounds the urethra; it grows with age, tightening on the urethra and making up for the weakening of the pelvic floor muscles with age. In benign enlargement of the prostate, this can be beneficial, but in other cases, prostate enlargement can create bacterial problems, discharge, and other more severe issues.

Pelvic Floor Exercises: Basics

Practicing pelvic floor exercises daily strengthens the muscles of the pelvic region and stimulates healthy blood flow. Strengthening the pelvic region, including the muscles of the urethra, vagina, and anus, improves pelvic health in general. It prevents or improves conditions of urinary or bowel incontinence and enhances sexual satisfaction. In addition, a daily practice will encourage health of the entire reproductive system; help prevent a prolapsed uterus or prolapsed bladder; reduce the risk of hemorrhoids, especially during pregnancy and childbirth; and, for pregnant women, help prevent tears in the perineum during delivery. Pelvic floor exercises aid in postpartum recovery. Pelvic floor exercises also ease the transition into menopause and maintain female health into older age. The practice of Pelvic Yoga is the integration of yoga postures with pelvic floor exercises for maximum improvement in pelvic floor strength and health.

Dr. Arnold Kegel developed Kegel exercises, which are also known as pelvic floor exercises. Pelvic floor exercises focus on toning the deep internal muscles of the pelvis. The technique improves bladder/bowel control, sexual response and functioning, and strength and tone of the pelvic and abdominal area. Pelvic exercises can also be a useful preventative health technique for high-risk populations, such as pregnant women, men with prostate problems, and persons with medical problems associated with risk of incontinence. In traditional Chinese medicine, pelvic floor exercises utilize the "jade gate." Qigong theory indicates pelvic floor exercises as useful for boosting health, especially for new mothers and women suffering from inhibited orgasm.

Pelvic Floor Exercises for Women

In women, the muscles isolated in pelvic floor exercises are shaped like a figure eight with the bulbospongiosus curving in front around the vaginal opening and urethra, crossing at the perineal body to meet the external sphincter ani, which curves back around the anus. When you perform pelvic floor exercises, you will feel a tightening of the entire figure eight, contracting the urethra, the vagina, and the anus. In the beginning of your practice, you may feel only one part of the muscles contracting. The contraction of the anus is the muscle action used to hold in gas or hold back a bowel movement. The contraction of the urethra is the muscle action used to hold in urine or to stop the flow during urination. The contraction of the vagina involves both the sphincter, which keeps it closed, and the folded muscles within the vaginal walls. Contracting the vaginal muscles during sexual intercourse and asking your sex partner for feedback is an effective technique for gaining control over the vaginal muscle. Eventually, you will develop your pelvic floor exercise technique for a full contraction of the entire figure eight. Some pelvic floor exercise techniques recommend dividing the exercise into three separate components—performing vaginal squeezes, anal squeezes, and urethral squeezes. While this is also a valid technique, it is easier and just as effective to work the entire figure eight at one time, rather than attempting to divide it into its components. As you develop body awareness of your pelvic region, you will become more adept at controlling the muscle movements throughout the figure eight.

The pelvic floor region, where the perineum is located, is shaped like a diamond with the top point formed by the pubic bone, or the symphysis pubis, and the bottom point formed by the tailbone, or the coccyx. The urethra, vagina, and rectum lie along the midline of this diamond. The muscles of the pelvic floor have to be strengthened around a "figure eight." The figure eight circles forwards around the vagina and urethra, crossing at the perineal body, and then backwards around the rectum. Pelvic floor exercises use the entire figure eight to strengthen the muscles throughout the pelvic region.

When you perform a pelvic floor exercise, close your rectum (as if preventing a bowel movement), draw the vagina in and up (as if gripping a tampon), and then tighten the urethra (as if stopping the flow of urine). When all three sections are contracted evenly, you have performed one pelvic floor exercise. Next, slowly and with control, release one section at a time—first the urethra, then the vagina, and finally the rectum. Then, release further, letting go of any residual tension in your pelvic muscles.

Pelvic Floor Exercises for Men

Pelvic floor exercises can help men strengthen the pelvic floor and increase or reestablish urinary control, even in the case of an enlarged prostate. In men, the figure eight is not quite a figure eight. The front muscle surrounds the shaft of the lower penis; the back muscle surrounds the rectum; and the center point is crossed at the perineal body. Pelvic floor exercises engage the entire not-quite-figure-eight, strengthening the muscles throughout the pelvic region. For men, the exercises involve the contraction of the rectum, as if suppressing gas, and the contraction of the urethra, as if stopping the flow of urine. A properly executed male pelvic floor exercise should include a slight movement of the penile head and a small lifted feeling at the perineal body.

When you perform a pelvic floor exercise, close your rectum (as if preventing a bowel movement), and then use the penile muscles to lift the penis and tighten the urethra (as if stopping the flow of urine). With a full contraction of this area, you have performed one repetition. Next, slowly and with control, release. Then, release further, letting go of any residual tension in your pelvic muscles. For men the strongest feel of the contraction will be in the rectum, and when done correctly, you will feel the rectum pull inward.

Three Techniques to Recognize Your Pelvic Muscles:

(1)   Stop Test

The Stop Test should only be done until you can recognize your pelvic muscles. Stopping urination is not healthy because it can snap bacteria into the urinary tract and can interfere with the bladder emptying mechanism. Do not try the Stop Test if you have a urinary tract or kidney infection. Never do the Stop Test more than once per day. If you are unable to stop urinating in the middle of the flow, do not get discouraged. With repeated effort, you will develop the body awareness to isolate the correct muscles.

To locate the pelvic floor, men should try the Stop Test. Like women, men should sit for this exercise. Standing while urinating will create muscular tension in the legs, making it more difficult to isolate the pelvic floor muscles. To perform this test:

- Sit on the toilet.

- Start urinating.

- Towards the end of the flow, try to stop urinating for one to two seconds. Completely relax. The muscles stopping the flow are the pelvic muscles. Learn to feel these muscles. Then finish urinating, completely emptying the bladder. The muscles you should focus on are the ones you feel squeezing around your urethra and anus.

- Practice squeezing these muscles when you are not urinating.

(2) Finger Test

Finger Test for Women

- Sit on a chair or lie down.
- Insert one or two fingers into the vagina.
- Squeeze and contract, as though you were holding back a bowel movement, lifting the vaginal walls up into the pelvic cavity. You should be able to feel the muscles tighten around your fingers.

Finger Test for Men

- Sit on a chair or lie down.
- Place your fingertip at the perineum, which is located between the base of the penis and the anus.
- Squeeze and contract, as though you were holding back a bowel movement. You should be able to feel the muscles lift away from your fingers. The penis should move slightly.

Alternatively, you can insert one finger into your rectum to test anal muscle strength.

(3) Medical Exam

Another technique for women is to ask your doctor during your next gynecological exam to test you for pelvic strength and rate you on a scale of one through ten (one weakest, ten strongest). With the doctor's fingers inside you, contract your pelvic muscles and hold.

Once you've identified the muscles, try placing the flat of your palm over the midline of your pelvic region with your pubic bone centered under the palm and the fingers over the vaginal cavity (for women) or on the perineum (for men). As you contract the pelvic floor muscles, you should feel a gentle "lift" of your pelvic muscles out of your hand. This will help you learn the feeling of isolating your pelvic floor muscles.

Pelvic Floor Exercise Tips

In the beginning, perform pelvic floor exercises while lying down on your back or side to learn to recognize the muscles and perform the actions correctly. Place the flat of your palm on your stomach, thigh, or buttocks. Focus your attention on the muscles under your hand, maintaining relaxation of that muscle. Clear any effort from the stomach, thighs, and buttocks, contracting only the pelvic floor muscles while relaxing the rest of your body. At first, practice your pelvic floor exercises lying on your back—completely relaxed—to facilitate the relaxation of stomach, thighs, and buttocks. Practice doing pelvic floor exercises in front of a mirror to ensure you have no abdominal movement.

With practice, you can learn to do these exercises while sitting, squatting, standing, or walking. When you are fully aware of the muscles and proper technique, add the pelvic exercises into your yoga routine for greater benefits.

Learn to integrate pelvic floor exercises into your daily life. For instance, you can use them while driving to work, standing in line at the grocery store, typing at your computer, cooking dinner, talking on the phone, or while showering. No one but you will know you are doing them. If the person next to you can see you move because you have contracted your stomach, thighs, or buttocks, you are doing the pelvic floor exercise incorrectly. Practice again while lying down to learn isolation of the pelvic floor muscles.

It is important to rest between each repetition of pelvic floor exercise for as long as you hold. Whenever you hold a pelvic floor contraction for five seconds, relax for at least five seconds. You must learn to completely "let go" and relax the pelvic muscles. Holding residual tension will weaken the pelvic floor and aggravate problems.

For the best long-term results, perform ninety repetitions per day. Do a combination of the exercises, spreading them out over three sessions of thirty repetitions or two sessions of forty-five repetitions each day. Less than ninety per day yields significantly less improvement, and more than ninety per day does not provide sufficiently greater improvement to merit the extra work. Ninety per day is the ideal program. Combine the different types of pelvic floor exercises into your Pelvic Yoga routine, rather than doing ninety repetitions of one type. Use a combination of slow and fast lifts. Perform repetitions of each of the advanced pelvic floor exercises (described later in this chapter, including Contract-Releases, Quick-Flicks, Long Holds, and Elevators). Supplement your Pelvic Yoga practice with Pelvic Yoga support practice to strengthen legs, abdominal muscles, hips, and lower back, thus supporting the entire pelvic region and encouraging better health in general. It is especially important to include the abdominal exercises for pelvic floor support.

Do your pelvic floor exercises each day in a variety of postures and positions. Seated practice strengthens your muscles when you are sitting. Standing practice strengthens your muscles when you are standing. Practice while lying down strengthens your muscles when you are lying down. Balance these exercises to balance your strength and holding ability. In the beginning, as you develop pelvic floor strength, practice while lying down to develop body awareness and strength. As you progress in your practice, add sitting and standing exercises. Eventually, add squats and inversions to further challenge your pelvic floor muscles and develop greater strength.

Pelvic health and pelvic floor strength requires a lifetime commitment. For long-term results, you have to do the exercises permanently, diligently, and on a daily basis. Learn to integrate them into your daily life—and your daily yoga practice—to facilitate this process. Making Pelvic Yoga practice a regular part of your exercise routine will increase fitness of the body while encouraging pelvic strength. You can develop two muscle tones for the time and effort of one.

Mistakes to Avoid

There are several common mistakes made while practicing pelvic floor exercises. Be careful to avoid the following:

- Do not hold your breath. This strains and pushes down instead of pulling up. You want to pull the pelvic muscles upwards into the cavity of your pelvis.

- Do not contract your abdominals.
- Do not contract your inner thighs.
- Do not contract your buttocks.

Four Advanced Pelvic Floor Exercise Techniques

(1) Contract-Release

The Contract-Release technique is the basic pelvic floor exercise. For women it is the most effective way to learn the feel of your pelvic floor muscles and develop muscular control over your urethral, vaginal, and anal sphincter. For men it is the most important way to gain control of the urethra, penis, and anus. Practice with Contract-Release to develop body awareness. To perform the Contract-Release technique:

- Contract and draw your pelvic floor up.
- Hold for five seconds.
- Relax completely.
- Relax even more, releasing residual tension. Rest five seconds.
- Repeat ten times per session, three sessions per day.

(2) Quick-Flicks

Quick-Flicks are like a "pelvic floor sprint." It is difficult to learn the "instantly contract" and then "instantly release" motions of the Quick-Flick. Generally, the body holds onto residuals of muscle tension, which are hard to release. Learning to move the pelvic floor in the rapid motion of the Quick-Flick helps to fine-tune your pelvic muscular control. To do a Quick-Flick:

- Tighten your pelvic floor, pulling up and in.
- Hold for only one to two seconds.
- Quickly release, relaxing completely. Rest one to two seconds.
- Repeat ten times per session, three times per day.

(3) Long Holds

Long Holds are the most important exercise for maintaining strength. In the beginning, Long Holds are difficult. Your pelvic floor muscles will weaken at approximately three seconds, six seconds, and nine seconds. As you feel your pelvic contraction start to drop, "re-grab" it and pull the muscles up and in. Slowly develop the endurance to hold Long Holds, which are the marathon of pelvic floor exercise. Work up to ten times per session, three times per day. To perform this exercise:

- Tighten your pelvic floor, pulling up and in.
- Hold for at least eight to ten seconds.
- Relax completely. Rest eight to ten seconds.

(4) Elevators

Elevators are time-consuming and difficult. At first, you will be unable to feel the distinction between four floors. It is common to feel only two floors when you begin. It is easier to climb through the floors than it is to descend through the floors with control. In the beginning, you will "lose" your tension as you descend. It is also difficult to hold tension at level four because your muscles will be very tired by that point. However, through Elevators you will see the greatest improvement in your pelvic floor strength and control. Elevators combine the fine-tuned muscular control of Quick-Flicks with the marathon-like endurance of Long Holds. Elevators are the hardest pelvic floor exercise to achieve, but they bring the greatest benefits.

Elevator training is also extremely important for individuals dealing with incontinence. Level two will become your "normal" level for bladder/pelvic control during sneezing, coughing, laughing, jumping, and exercising. Once you have learned the feel of level two and can contract your pelvic muscles directly to the second floor, you can use the technique to prevent incidents of incontinence. Before sneezing, laughing, coughing, jumping, or performing any activity that may normally cause urine leaking, elevate your pelvic floor to level two (remembering the four floors from the Elevator). Relax, breathe, and calm yourself. Gain control. Then contract and hold at level two during the activity. Do not attempt to hold at level four, as you will drop the contraction and perhaps leak. Level two can be held throughout an activity and will help prevent urinary leakage. To perform Elevators:

Imagine your pelvis has four floors.

- Contract, pulling your pelvic muscles up gently to floor one. Hold the tension.

- Contract, holding the tension of floor one and pulling up a little farther to floor two. Hold.

- Contract, holding floor two and pulling up to floor three. Hold.

- Contract, holding floor three and pulling up to floor four. Hold.

- Contract and hold at floor four.

- Slowly, relax down through the floors, one by one.

- Relax, holding some of the tension but releasing down to floor three. Hold.

- Relax, holding some of the tension but releasing down to floor two. Hold.

- Relax, holding some of the tension but releasing down to floor one. Hold.

- Relax down to the "basement," completely letting go.

- Rest ten seconds.

- Repeat ten times per session, three times per day.

Pelvic Yoga—an Integrated Program of Pelvic Floor Exercise

Integrating pelvic floor rehabilitation exercise with a well-designed yoga practice is the most efficient way to strengthen and improve the health of your pelvic floor. In the beginning, the pelvic floor exercises will be difficult to perform while holding yoga postures. With diligent daily practice, you will develop the strength and capability to perform ninety repetitions per day as part of your yoga regime. When beginning poses become simple, progress to moderate postures. Moderate and advanced yoga postures assume a certain level of yoga proficiency and practice. Beginning yoga students should maintain their Pelvic Yoga practice utilizing the beginning poses. Until you can perform the moderate and advanced poses comfortably, you are not ready to integrate the pelvic floor exercises into those poses. If your body is tense and the yoga posture is uncomfortable or strained, it is impossible to relax sufficiently to perform an effective pelvic floor contraction. An important thing to remember is that in yoga everything should be steady and comfortable (according to Patanjali's *Yoga Sutras,* which is the classical yoga text). Stop if you have pain or feel strained, if your breath becomes difficult, or if you feel uneasy or unhappy. Remember, yoga should be comfortable!

Yoga Breath

Breathwork is an integral part of yoga. Feel your body and movements flowing with your breath, as if your body were a raft on the river of your breath. In general, inhale as you move up, expand, open, and stretch. In general, exhale as you move down, contract within, and twist. In terms of breathwork, integrate the general principles—expanding, lifting, reaching, opening—when you inhale. When you exhale, use the following principles: contracting, bending, closing, and twisting. The simplest rule is that if you are moving in a way that creates more space in your abdomen—by lifting the ribs or stretching open the chest—inhale to fill that space. If you are moving in a way that lessens the space in your abdomen—by bending forward, twisting, or closing down the front of your body—exhale to create more space. Breathe fully and deeply, reaching into the diaphragm to completely fill the lungs. Shallow chest breathing constricts movement; work to expand your lungs and breathe to enhance flowing movement. Integrate the general breath principles into your thoughts and understanding. Then flow, allowing your breath to happen naturally.

Yoga Vision

Where to look is another issue of consequence, in shaping a yoga practice. Again, flow with your instincts. In balance poses like Tree, finding a focal point in the distance can provide stability. In sitting poses and inversions, closing your eyes helps create a greater sense of peace. By closing your eyes in a yoga posture and going within to find your center, you can open your eyes to life anew, looking at the world with clear vision, seeing the life and answers you need. While the practice of yoga does not change the world, it changes your heart.

Pelvic Floor Exercise and Yoga Bandhas ("Locks")

The yoga bandhas, or locks, are lifts of the lower chakras to raise the Kundalini energy up the spine. Kundalini is the life force energy, and it is parallel to Qi / Ki / Chi in Chinese theory. Kundalini fills your body and determines your health and vitality. It begins in the first chakra (the root chakra), which is located at the perineum. This sexually toned energy can be charged and channeled up the spine to become a spiritual energy, which increases vitality. Kundalini, which also means *snake,* is "wound up" the spine into the higher chakras, like a snake coiling up the body. According to Shakti Parwha Kaur Khalsa, as taught by Yogi Bhajan, you can improve your mood and your spirits by raising your Kundalini energy.

In Ashtanga yoga theory, the locks, or Bandhas, are a series of internal energy gates, which assist in the regulation of pranic flow. They are valves. Just as circulatory valves keep blood flowing through the veins and arteries, preventing backwash, the locks keep the subtle energy of the body, or prana, moving through the energetic channels, or nadis. Using the locks, we force energy through the nadis and revitalize our bodies.

Ashtanga Yoga Root Lock

Ashtanga yoga master David Swenson uses the Kegel exercise technique to teach Root Lock, or Mulabandha. He says that you can practice Mulabandha by contracting the anus, and that it is subtle like the Kegel technique. Mulabandha is called Root Lock because of its location at the base of our nerve tree, which in yoga theory is considered the root. For men, Mulabandha is activated at the perineal muscle, between the anus and the genitals. For women, Mulabandha is near the top of the cervix.

Root Lock is maintained throughout the duration of a ninety-minute Ashtanga yoga practice session. In the beginning of Ashtanga Root Lock work, it is impossible to hold Mulabandha throughout your practice. Whenever you drop it, pick it up again and continue with the practice. As pelvic floor strength and control increase, work to hold Mulabandha throughout the duration of your Ashtanga yoga session.

Kundalini Energy

According to Kundalini yoga theory, if energy remains in the lower chakras, these chakras control us and we suffer. However, we can re-channel the lower energy into the higher consciousness of the upper chakras; for instance, the fire energy can be transformed into courage and initiative. The Root Lock closes off the lower chakras, which forces the Kundalini energy to flow upward. Critical to the channeling of Kundalini energy is a straight and healthy spine, so that energy can freely flow up the spinal cord. Yoga theorists caution that the practice of Root Lock is an advanced spiritual practice for which we must appropriately prepare, via yoga and meditation practice.

Root Lock

The Root Lock, known as the Mul Bandh in Kundalini Yoga and Mulabandha in

Ashtanga Yoga, is the lock of the first root, or chakra. It is very similar to a pelvic floor exercise. The Kundalini method to performing Root Lock is as follows:

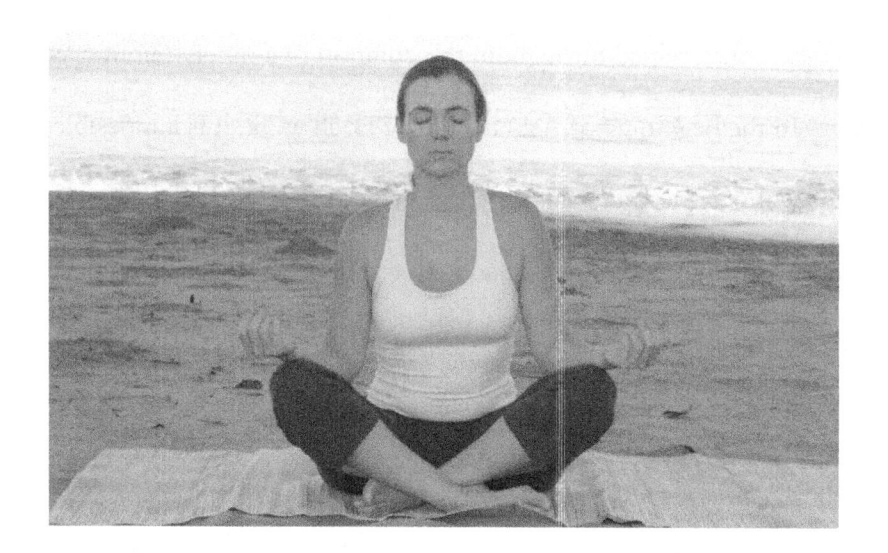

- Sit in a comfortable, cross-legged position.

- Inhale as deeply as possible, lifting your chest but keeping yours shoulders relaxed away from your ears.

- Exhale, releasing your breath fully while keeping your chest lifted.

- With your body empty of breath, contract the muscles of your rectum, sex organ (vagina in women, penis in men), and navel point (at your belly button). Pull your navel in and up. Hold.

- Inhale. Relax the contraction.

- Repeat, practicing for several minutes.

Sat Kriya

Kundalini practice uses Mul Bandh in several postures. Sat Kriya is the most powerful of the poses in which to practice Mul Bandh. Sat Kriya raises the Kundalini energy up the channel of the spine for greater vitality and life force. It should be practiced for three minutes per day, up to thirty-one minutes per day, with an equal amount of relaxation afterward. To perform Sat Kriya:

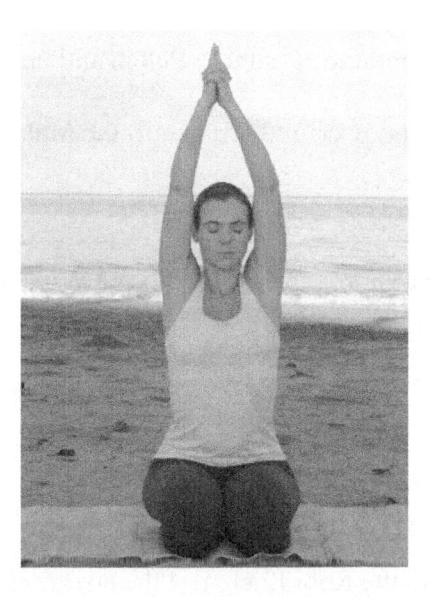

- Sit on your heels.
- Lift your arms over your head. Touch your palms together with fingers interlaced, index fingers pointed toward the sky, upper arms pressed into your ears, and arms held perfectly straight.

- Close your eyes, focusing your attention on the third-eye-point between your brows. This point is an important spiritual point in yogic theory because it is the seat of intuition and wisdom. In physiological terms, the position of the third eye is in a line in front of the pineal and pituitary glands, which are located within the center area of the brain, behind the forehead. Therefore, it is possible that focusing the energy at the third eye point could stimulate functioning of the pineal and pituitary glands. Maintain this focus of your eyes throughout Sat Kriya.

- Inhale, chant SAT (pronounced "suht"). Pull in and up on your navel, lifting your arms with strength and power, and lifting into the Mul Bandh. Make a strong, solid sound.

- Release the lock with a short exhalation on NAAM (pronounce "nom.")

- Continue inhaling and contracting the Root Lock on SAT and exhaling and releasing on NAAM.

- At first, perform this move for one minute.

- Inhale, tightly contract the Root Lock, feel the energy channel up your spine, and hold for ten seconds.

- Exhale, release, and relax.

- Repeat two more times.

- Relax, release the arms down to your sides, sit with your eyes closed, and return to normal, relaxed breathing.

Root Lock During Menstruation

Kundalini theory cautions that menstruating women should not perform Root Lock, especially during the heavy portion of the flow. Many yoga theories advise against the practice of strenuous yoga during menstruation. However, some yoga theorists believe this is due to a lack of tradition for women in yoga. During the thousands of years of yoga's development in India, women were not allowed to practice yoga. Because of the release of body fluids during a woman's menstrual cycle, she was considered unclean. Therefore, when women began to practice yoga, and as yoga came to the West over the past century, it is possible that the precautions about avoiding yoga practice during menstruation were based more on prejudice and sexism than on energy or health. Some yoga teachers warn that a woman is more fragile and tires more easily during menstruation, which makes her incapable of strenuous yoga practice. Some yoga practitioners find that a strenuous yoga practice during the menstrual cycle can relieve tension, improve symptoms of mental discomfort, and lessen cramps. You know your own body best. Listen to the intuitive wisdom of your body for the answers to your questions.

Stomach Lock

Stomach Lock (also see Stomach Contractions in Section 3) can also assist with issues of incontinence by strengthening muscles in the lower abdomen. Practice two to three times per day and you will notice results within two to three weeks. Avoid stomach lock if you have high blood pressure, heart disease, a hernia, or if you are pregnant. To perform Stomach Lock:

- Lie on your back.
- Breathe in deeply.
- Breathe out completely, expelling every bit of air from your lungs.
- With no breath, contract your buttocks, groin, and stomach muscles powerfully and simultaneously.
- Hold for a count of three.
- Release.
- Repeat two more times.

Beginning Poses

(1) Simple Sitting Contract-Releases

Simple Sitting is a relaxed form of sitting cross-legged with awareness to maintain a straight spine. This can be a very natural, comfortable position. Initially, you can use simple sitting to practice all your pelvic floor exercises.

Pregnant women will find that sitting cross-legged opens up space for the expanding belly. With both legs on the floor, a balanced foundation creates support and comfort for the spine. Doing arm stretches in Simple Sitting—simply lifting the arms and chest toward the ceiling gently—is a good way to expand the abdominal cavity and create more space for the growing baby and womb. To do Simple Sitting Contract-Releases:

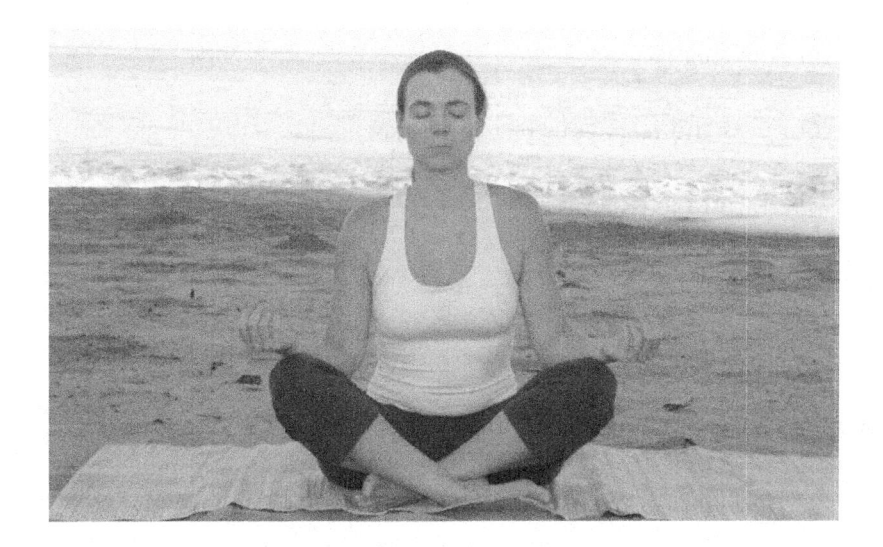

- Sit on the floor, crossing your legs loosely and comfortably at about the shin. Tuck your feet under with feet and toes relaxed on the floor.

- Ground your sit bones into the floor, feeling the solid foundation of your lower body. Use your hands to pull the flesh out from underneath your bottom, so that your sit bones firmly press into the flour. If necessary, you can put a bolster, pillow, or blanket under your buttocks to lift your hips. This will help you to maintain a straight spine and make your bottom more comfortable.

- Concentrate on your posture, maintaining a long spine and straight back. Relax your neck and tuck your chin in gently to lengthen the back of the neck. At the same time, lift the crown of your head toward the ceiling, making you feel tall. Align your head, neck, and trunk over the base of your spine.

- Your arms should be relaxed at the sides of the body with your hands resting with palms on your thighs.
- Close your eyes and relax your facial muscles.
- Perform ten Contract-Releases.
- Release and relax.

(2) Cat-Cow Pose Contract-Release

Because your pelvis tilts as you lift back and forth, the Cat-Cow pose is an effective posture to flow with Contract-Releases. Cat-Cow is good for opening up the bones of the pelvis and loosening tightness in the pelvic region. It is also an effective posture for preventing or working to overcome a dowager's hump. In the Cat-Cow pose, the shoulders roll back and the chest pulls through the upper arms, lifting. This stretches open the chest, counteracting the tightness across the middle back, which causes poor posture and stooping in older women.

Cat posture (Dromedary Droop) is useful throughout pregnancy and labor to relieve the pressure of an enlarged uterus on your spine. It also helps open the hips and pelvis to facilitate delivery. Kneeling on all fours is effective for relieving pregnancy-related backache because it takes weight off the lower back. To perform the Cat-Cow Pose Contract-Release:

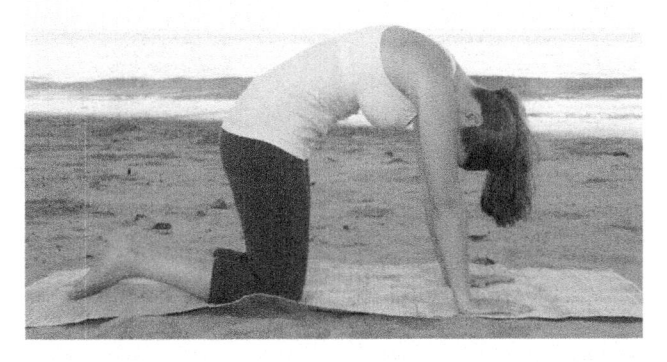

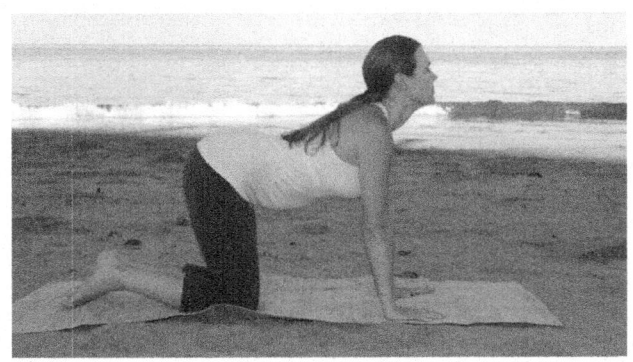

- Get on your hands and knees.

- Align your knees directly under your hips. Align to your actual hipbone, not the width of your hips based on spreading. The tops of your feet should be flat against the floor.

- Align your hands directly under your shoulders. Your middle fingers should be pointing forward with your thumbs facing each other. Press your weight evenly into the entire palm of the hand. Do not cup your palm because that places too much weight on your wrist.

- Your back and neck should be relaxed and comfortable.

- Exhaling, drop your chin into your neck while arching your spine like a cat. Contract your pelvic floor. Hold.

- Inhaling, lift your chin, lengthen your neck, and look at the ceiling while dropping your back down into the swayback position of a cow. Feel the bones of your pelvis spread open gently as you release the pelvic floor contraction. Rest.

- Repeat ten times.

(3) Child's Pose Quick-Flicks

Child's Pose is a wonderful yoga pose. It soothes the spine and the nervous system and relaxes the body. It also brings relaxation to the reproductive organs and is effective in alleviating menstrual cramps. It promotes circulation, facilitates elimination, and releases lower-back tension. After a strenuous yoga routine, this pose calms and heals. To do Child's Pose Quick-Flicks:

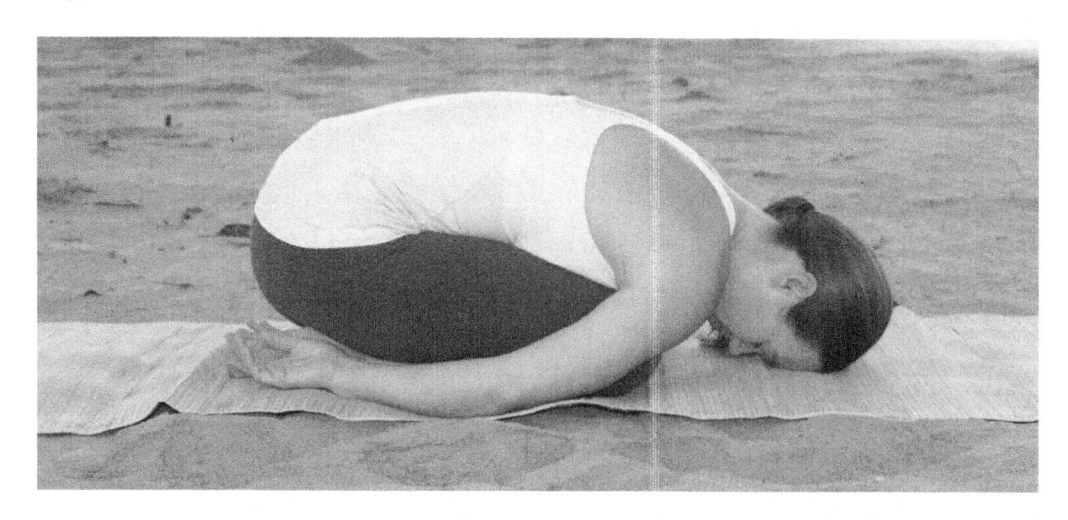

- Kneel with the tops of your feet flat on the floor. Sit back on your heels. If this is uncomfortable, place a blanket between your bottom and the tops of your calves to create space and make sitting back easier.
- Slowly and gently, bend your body at the waist. Rest your chest against your thighs. If you are tight and unable to reach your chest to your thighs, place a pillow on top of your thighs.
- Relax your neck muscles and release your head to the floor.
- Rest your arms along the side of your body with palms up.
- Resting in Child's Pose, repeat ten Quick-Flicks.
- Release Child's Pose by sitting up slowly and with control.

(4) Chair Quick-Flicks

The Chair Pose strengthens the legs, lower back, and abdomen, as you draw in the entire core of the body for balance and stability. Chair also uses the strength of the inner thighs, channeling energy throughout the pelvic region. As strength in the pose develops, and you are capable of sitting lower in Chair while maintaining a straight back, the focus of muscular effort on the pelvis continues to expand and increase, strengthening the entire pelvic region. Performing pelvic floor exercises while in Chair is a synergistic posture with the efforts of the pelvic floor exercise reinforcing the efforts of the Yoga Posture, and vice versa. To perform the Chair Quick-Flicks:

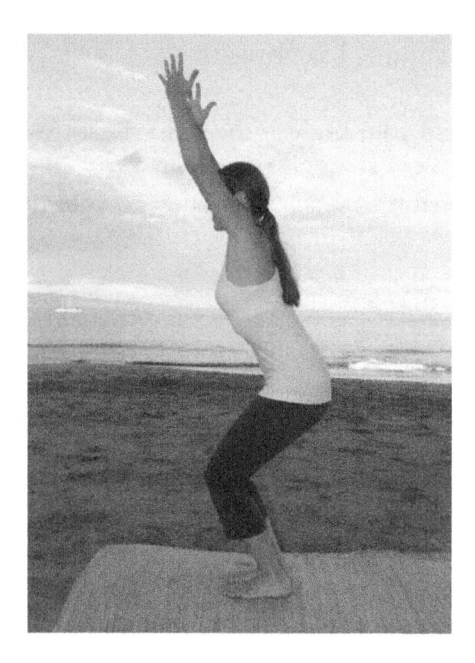

- Stand with your feet together, toes touching, heels slightly parted, weight centered over the arches of your feet. Tuck your tailbone under and draw your abdomen in; press your knees and ankles together; roll your shoulders down the back, releasing your arms loosely at the sides of the body.

- Inhale. Lift your arms up until your palms touch over your head. Keep your arms straight and lifted. Do not lift your shoulders.

- While stretching and lifting the chest, tilt your chin and look up at your fingertips.

- Exhale, while keeping your arms lifted. Bend your knees and slide down into the Chair Pose. Make sure to keep your lower back and abdomen tucked into the core of your body. If this posture is uncomfortable, start with your feet about one to two feet from the wall, slide down the wall into Chair, pressing your back into the wall for support.

- Holding Chair, perform ten Quick-Flicks.

- To release, inhale while standing up. Release the tension in your legs while still looking up.

- Exhale. Release your arms to your sides and relax.

(5) Staff Pose with Long Holds

Staff Pose seems to be an easy posture, but when practiced with diligent awareness, it requires effort and focus. Staff Pose helps you gain awareness of the proper alignment of your pelvis and spine, teaching you the proper sitting position. To perform the Staff Pose with Long Holds:

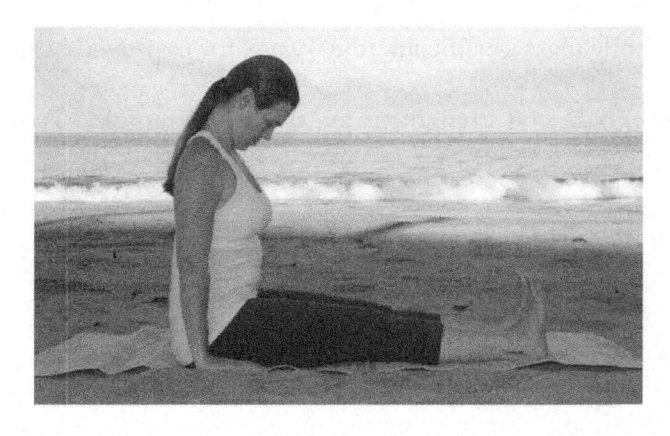

- Sit on the floor with your legs together and straight in front of you. Pull your toes back toward your face. Then lift the balls of your feet toward the ceiling, while grounding your heels into the floor. Activate your thigh muscles, pressing the backs of your knees into the floor.
- Place your hands on each side of your hips with your palms firmly pressed into the ground. Use the strength of your arms to straighten your upper body and lift your spine without artificially lifting your shoulders to your ears.
- Breathe deeply, keeping your body relaxed but active.
- Perform ten Long Holds.
- Relax and release.

(6) Wind-Relieving Pose with Long Holds

The Wind-Relieving Pose relieves digestive wind. The posture helps with gas, constipation, diarrhea, and other digestive disorders. The pressure of the knee into the abdominal cavity gently massages the internal organs for improved health. It also relieves pressure in the lower back and strengthens the abdominal muscles. To do this move:

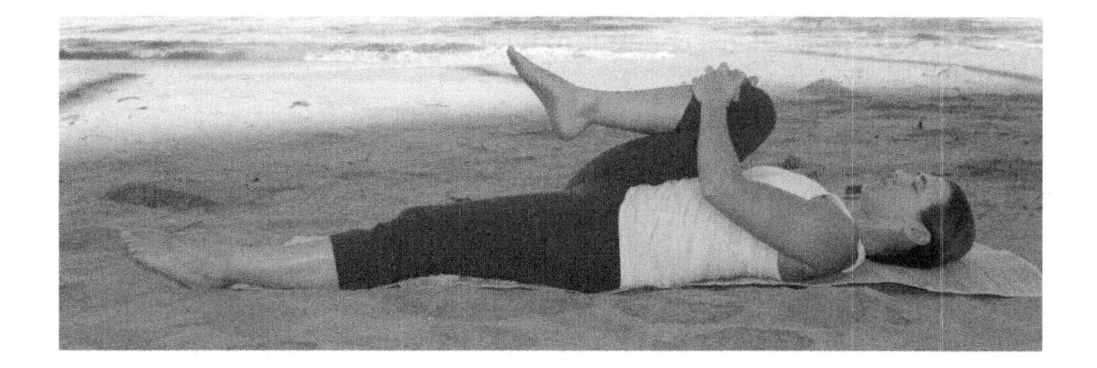

- Lie flat on your back with your legs relaxed and your head and neck comfortably resting on the ground. (Use a small blanket or pillow under your head, if that is more comfortable). Inhale deeply.

- Exhale, lifting your right knee into your chest, pointing your toe, wrapping your arm around the outside of the knee, and then pulling your thigh into your body. Maintain the integrity of your left leg by firmly pressing it into the floor with your foot flexed and toes drawing back toward your face.

- Perform a Long Hold, remembering to breathe.

- Relax, and then release your right leg to the floor.

- Inhale deeply.

- Exhale, lifting your left knee into your chest, pointing your toe, wrapping your arm around the outside of the knee, and then pulling your thigh into your body. Maintain the integrity of your right leg by firmly pressing it into the floor with your foot flexed and toes drawing back toward your face.

- Perform a Long Hold, remembering to breathe.

- Relax, and then release your left leg to the floor.

- Repeat for ten Long Holds.

(7) Mountain Pose Balance with Elevators

Mountain Pose is deceptively simple. A balanced, calm Mountain Pose requires full mental concentration. It helps to establish a sense of one's balance and calms the entire body. It quiets the mind and centers the spirit.

Elevators are very difficult to do. Until you have achieved "Elevator Proficiency," use Mountain Pose and Corpse Pose for Elevator practice. You will feel the difference in your balance as you do Mountain Pose Balance with Elevator; your body will feel off-centered and probably sway. Do not be shocked by this. It is challenging to maintain your balance while focusing on your pelvic floor muscles.

To do the Mountain Pose with Elevators:

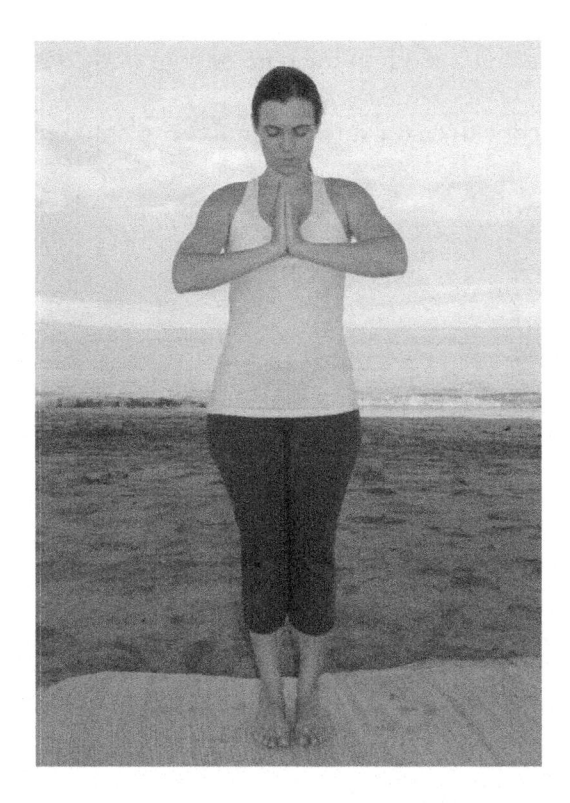

- Stand with your feet together, toes touching, heels slightly apart, and your body weight centered over your arches.

- Pose with your palms together, centered between your breasts, and your upper arms gently relaxed.

- Activate your upper thigh muscles by lifting them into the hips to strengthen and tone, as well as to protect your knees.

- Your spine should be long and fluid. Your neck should be long and relaxed with your chin tucked in slightly to open up the back of your neck.

- Tuck your tailbone and torso into the core of your body. Feel how your body is strong and balanced with a straight spine and feet planted firmly on the ground.
- Perform ten Elevators.

(8) Corpse Pose Elevator

Corpse Pose, or Sponge Pose, is the hardest of all yoga postures. Although it is physically simple, it requires a great deal of mental energy and effort. When lying on your back, you may fall asleep. Focusing energy and channeling awareness to remain fully aware requires great patience and calm. Corpse Pose balances the nervous system, restores energy, and calms the mind. It also puts less strain on the heart by dropping the entire body to the same level.

Corpse is a good posture in which to learn Elevator because the pelvic region is relaxed and gravity has minimal impact. Begin your Elevator practice with daily Corpse Pose work until you know your Elevator and your pelvic muscles well enough to practice in different postures and situations. To perform the Corpse Pose Elevator:

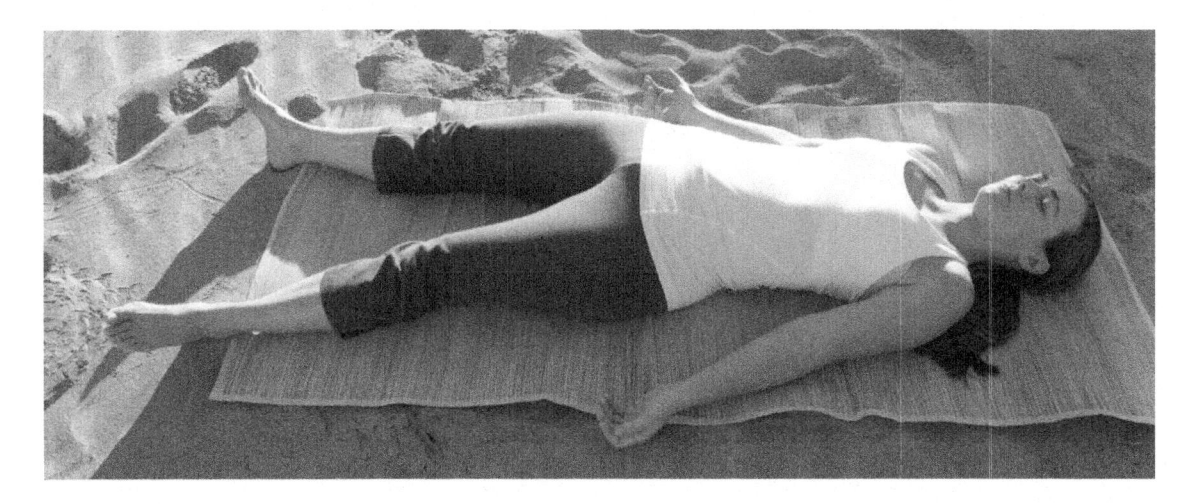

- Lying flat on your back, release completely and melt into the floor.

- Place your hands with your palms facing up about six inches to one foot away from each thigh.

- Spread your legs with feet hip width apart.

- If your head is uncomfortable, use a small pillow under your neck.

- If your lower back is strained, place a rolled blanket or pillow under your knees.

- Release the weight of your body into the floor, feeling the tension dissolve. Make sure the full length of your spine is pressing into the ground. If your lower back is lifting, bend your knees and roll the spine into the floor slowly, vertebrae by vertebrae, to melt the entire length of the spine into the floor.

- Breathe deeply and regularly.

- Perform ten Elevators.

- When you are finished, release and relax.

Moderate Poses

(1) Perfect Posture Contract-Release (Tailor Pose)

This is a good posture for opening up the groin. Perfect Posture, or the Tailor Pose, is important for lower back and thigh health. It is also a good posture to practice during long periods of sitting. Perfect Posture improves or prevents sciatica, due to its gentle stretching of your hips. Perfect Posture is also beneficial to the entire pelvic region. To perform this pose:

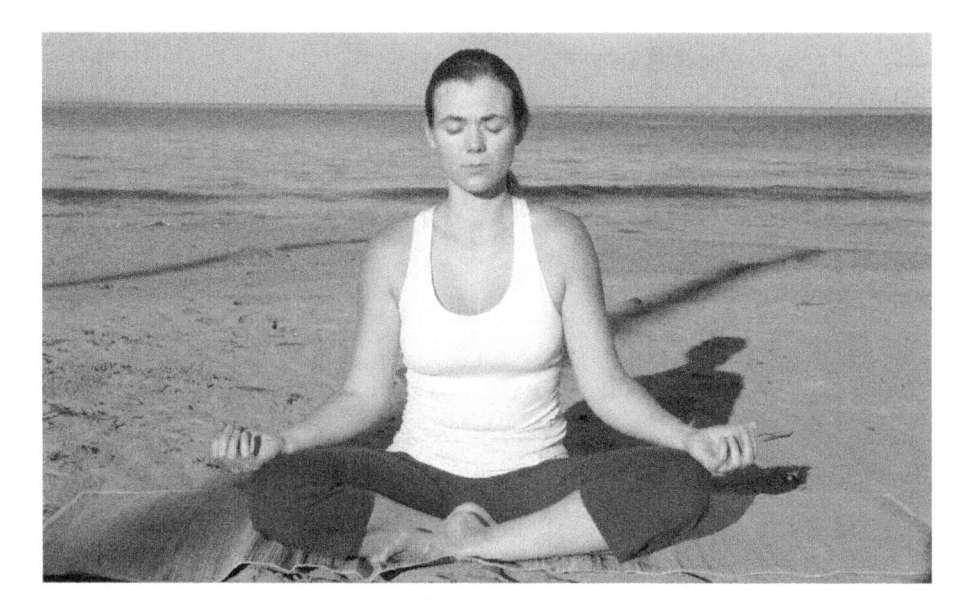

- Sit on a pillow, blanket, or zafu to lift your hips. This facilitates the proper alignment of your spine.

- Fold your legs and bring one heel into your groin with the bottom of the foot and toes gently rested along the opposite thigh.

- Fold your other leg, bringing the second heel in so that your heels are in a straight line from the groin. Your second foot should be placed so that the heels are almost (but not quite) stacked with the Achilles heel of your outside foot resting along the top of your inside foot.
- Rest your hands on your thighs with your palms up.
- Find a comfortable balance with your back straightened, spine relaxed, neck lengthened, muscles of the face softened, and your eyes closed.
- Breathe naturally and gently, while performing ten Contract-Releases.
- Relax, uncrossing your legs gently. Then release.

(2) Camel Contract-Release

Camel Posture is a powerful pose for opening up the pelvic region. It is a therapeutic posture, good for hips and thighs as well as the glands and nerves. Camel Pose also vitalizes your endocrine glands, such as the thyroid and ovaries, and strengthens the urinary and reproductive systems. Camel is a good posture for an active pelvic floor meditation. Lifting your hips takes them to the center of awareness, channeling energy to the pelvic region. In Camel, focus your energy on the pelvic region, feeling your blood and awareness flow to the core of your body. To perform the Camel Contract-Release:

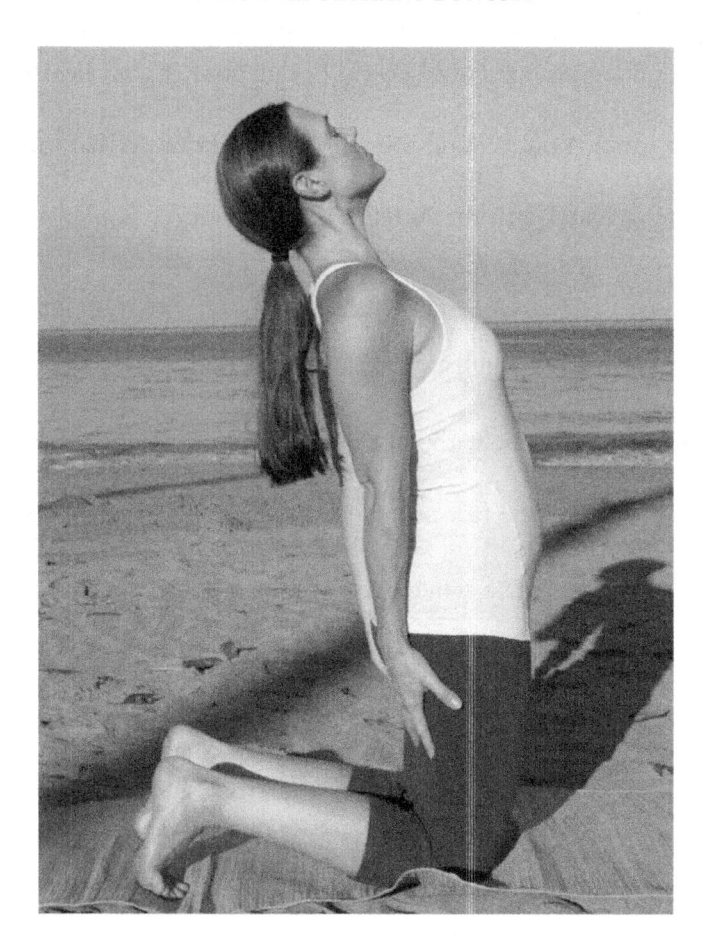

- Kneel on the floor with your knees directly under the hipbones.

- To begin, curl your toes, propping your heels into the air.

- Place the flat of your palm on the back of your upper thigh and lower buttocks.

- Roll your shoulders back gently, lifting forward through your chest. Tilt your chin toward the ceiling, and press the palms of your hands into your upper thighs to attain a gentle lift.

This is the first level of Camel. If you feel comfortable here, remain here. Breathing gently, perform ten Contract-Releases.

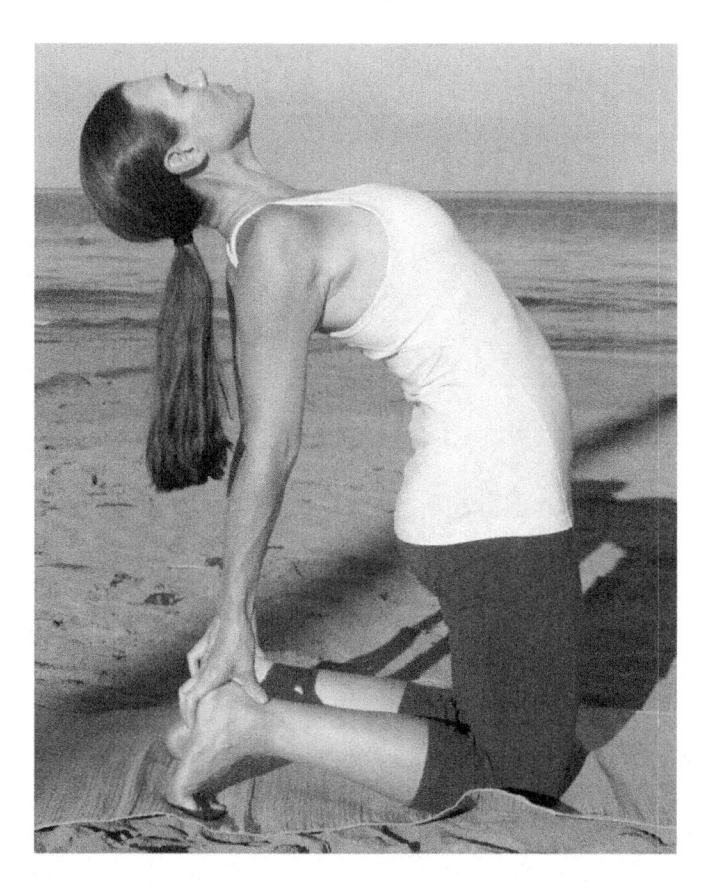

- Or, you can continue to the next level of Camel.

- Maintaining a straight line from your knee to hip (do not cave backwards), reach back with your right hand toward your raised right heel. If this is comfortable, take your left hand back toward your raised left heel.

- Holding onto your heels, lift forward and up, through the chest and chin to open the front of the body. Pull your weight forward, maintaining it in a straight line from knee to hip.

This is the second level of Camel. If you feel comfortable here, remain here. Breathing gently, perform ten Contract-Releases.

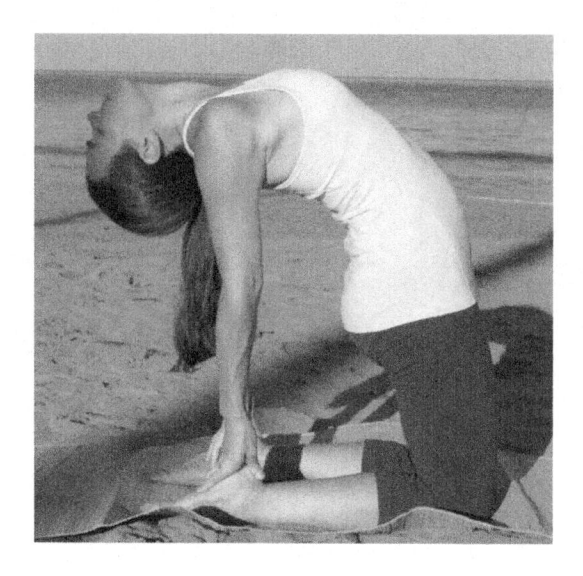

- Or, you can continue to the next level of Camel.

- Flatten the tops of your feet along the floor, holding onto your heels with your hands and continuing the lift and forward motion of your chest and chin. Your neck should drop back with your head resting between your shoulders.

- Breathing gently, perform ten Contract-Releases.

(3) Frog Pose Quick-Flicks

Frog Pose is beneficial for the lower back and hips. It can relieve (or at least lessen) sciatica pain and keep your sciatic nerves in better shape to prevent the recurrence of pain. It is also helpful for stretching a tight psoas muscle and opening up the pelvic region. To perform this pose:

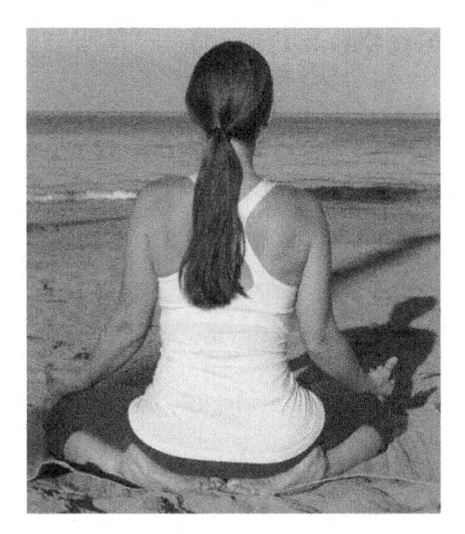

- Kneel down on the floor with your toes and feet touching.

- Spread your knees apart as wide as possible, respecting your comfort level but challenging yourself to stretch your inner thighs with a gentle, slow posture. Keep your toes touching behind your buttocks.

- Sit back against your feet. The arches will create a small "hammock" between your heels. Rest your bottom in that hammock. If this is uncomfortable, place a blanket, pillow, or bolster under your bottom so that you can sit without discomfort.

- Rest your hands on your knees.

- Breathe gently and naturally, performing ten Quick-Flicks.

- Relax and release.

- Use your hands to help draw your knees back together.

- Rest while sitting on your knees. Then slowly get up.

(4) Squatting, Legs Together, Quick-Flicks

Squatting—whether with your legs together or apart—is helpful for developing pelvic strength and control. In cultures where people regularly squat, they have stronger legs and healthier bowels. Squatting provides lower back support, massages abdominal muscles and organs, facilitates circulation, and prevents constipation.

Squatting takes practice to do it comfortably because our western legs are not used to the pelvic spread. Women considering pregnancy should practice squatting because it can help take the weight off the low back, even during delivery. However, squatting can be difficult. An experienced squatter will find herself having to readjust throughout pregnancy as her center of gravity changes; a new squatter may find the posture difficult to attempt if already pregnant. For best results, develop a comfortable squat before you get pregnant. To perform the Squatting Pose:

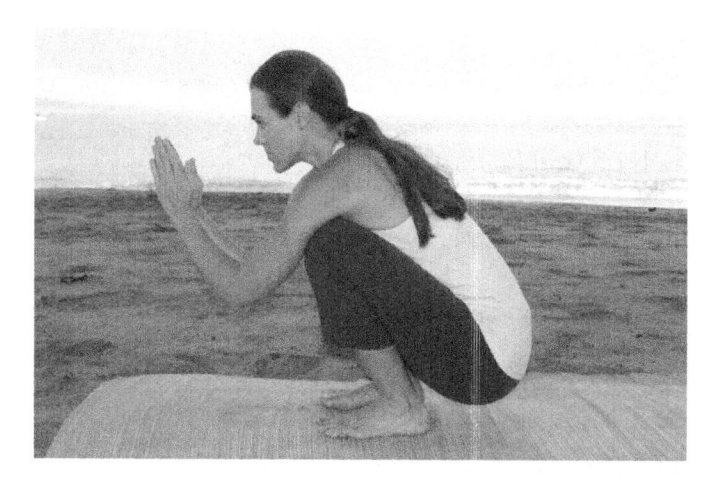

- Position yourself with your feet as close as possible, toes facing forward, and heels firmly grounded into the floor.

- Squat as low as you can. You will eventually want your heels to relax on the floor while you squat. In the beginning however, your calf muscles are tight, so your heels might remain lifted off the floor.

- Push the backs of your arms into your knees for balance with your knees coming into your armpits and your chest resting against your thighs.

- Make your back and spine as straight and long as possible. Keep your head and chin lifted. Find your center, and balance into the pose. (Alternatively, you can squat in front of a chair with your hands on the chair for support. You can also stand near a wall and squat, resting your back and buttocks against the wall for support. Do not strain yourself by overdoing.)

- Breathe and relax, performing ten Quick-Flicks.

(5) Squatting, Legs Apart, Elevator

For pregnancy, squatting with your legs apart is a critical element of a prenatal practice because it facilitates the spread of the pelvic bones. To perform Squatting, Legs Apart:

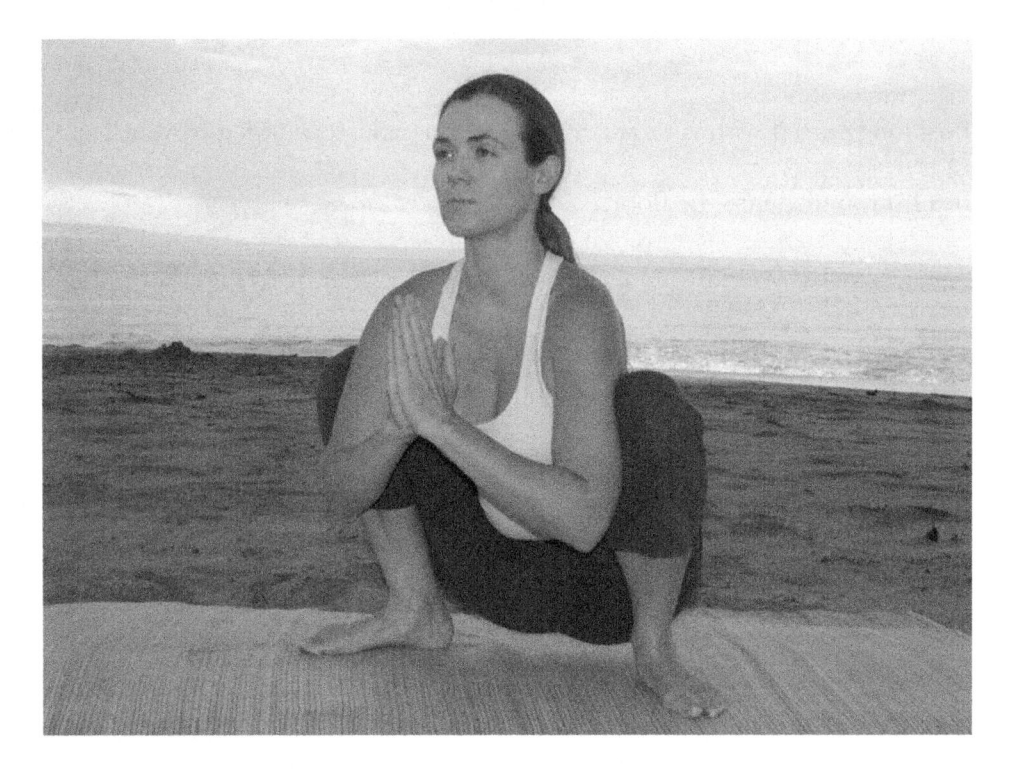

- Position yourself with your feet apart and your toes pointing outward.

- Squat, lowering your buttocks between your legs. If you need to, hold the back of a chair or position yourself against a wall for balance.

- Bring your hands together in Namaste, or prayer position, at your heart. Use your elbows to help balance by pushing against the inside of your thighs and knees and encouraging the necessary outward rotation.

- Find your center and balance in the pose. (When you first start practicing this pose, you can lower your buttocks to the floor for better balance, but make sure to keep your spine long and lifted, even as you lower your bottom to the floor.)

- Breathe and relax, performing ten Elevators.

(6) Cobbler's Pose Elevators

Like Squatting, Legs Apart, Cobbler's Pose opens up the groin, hips, and pelvis. Do not push down on your knees in an attempt to force your inner thighs open. This can lead to injury, especially to your knees. Instead, use your feet. Place your fingers around the outside of your foot with the thumb pressing into the center bottom. Firmly yet gently, pull open your feet. This will create more space, facilitating your hips to open. Over time, your knees will fall open naturally without force or injury. To perform Cobbler's Pose:

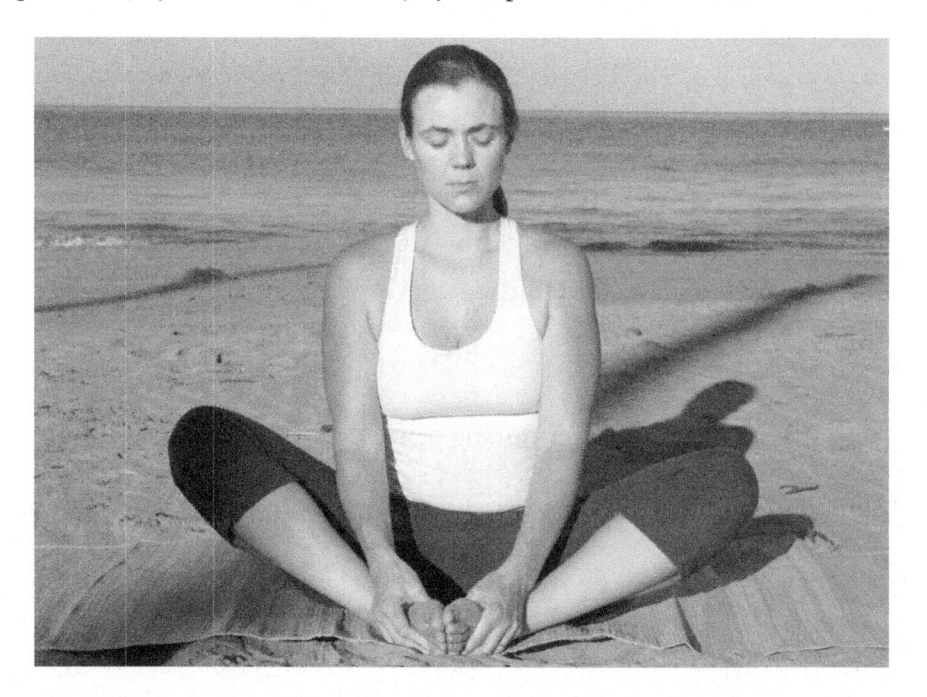

- Sit on the floor. Place a blanket, pillow, or bolster under your hips if you need a little lift to maintain a straight spine.

- Bring the soles of your feet together, sliding your heels in toward the groin.

- Hold your feet in your hands with your fingers wrapped around the top of each foot and your thumb pressing into the bottom center of each foot. Use your hands to open your feet, which will, in turn, gently open your hips.

- Press your elbows into your thighs, simultaneously pushing open your thighs and knees with your elbows while pulling your chest forward to lift and open.

- Keep your sit bones grounded into the floor with your spine lifted and long and your body relaxed.

- Breathing gently and naturally, perform ten Elevators.

- Relax. Use your hands to help release your legs. Sit for a moment with your legs in front of you to release any tension in the inner thighs.

(7) Tree Pose Balance with Long Holds

Tree Pose helps to cultivate a sense of internal peace and balance. Tree also stretches and strengthens the pelvis and legs. Performing pelvic floor exercise while in Tree is an ultimate challenge of balance, pushing you to utilize your muscles and concentration to hold the pose while having freedom of thought and effort to perform pelvic floor exercise. To do Tree Pose Balance with Long Holds:

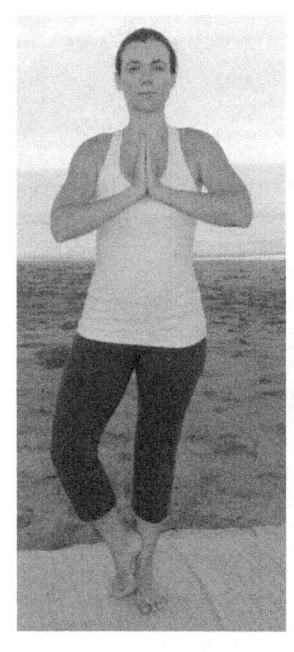

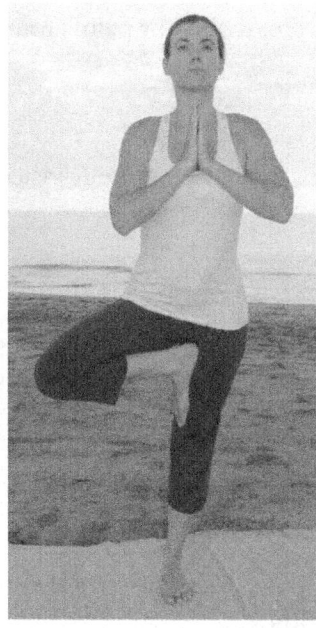

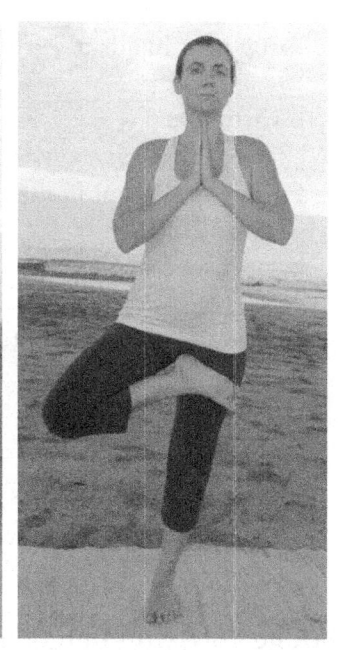

- Begin in Mountain Pose with your feet together, toes touching, and heels slightly parted. Balance your weight evenly over the arches of your foot. Tuck in your tailbone and your abdominal muscles, centering the core of your body.

- From Mountain Pose, shift your weight to the left foot. Calmly, balancing gently and with lightness, lift your right foot. Balance the foot on the ankle of the left leg. If this feel comfortable and you would like to increase the difficulty of the pose, use your right hand to bring the sole of the right foot up to the inside of your left thigh (moderate) or into your groin area (advanced). Finding your balanced center, hold the posture. Keep your standing leg slightly bent to protect your knee. Rotate the right thigh outward to open up the hip.

- Bring your hands to Namaste, with your palms touching, centered over your breastbone.

- Find a focal point in the distance. Center your vision on this point to increase balance and stability.

- Perform five Long Holds, breathing throughout.

- Relax. Lower your leg.

- Repeat on the opposite side.

(8) Bridge Pose with Long Holds

Bridge Pose is effective for increasing flexibility of the pelvic region while developing subtle control of the low back, abdomen, and thighs. Be careful with your neck in Bridge Pose. Never turn your head while holding Bridge Pose. Always maintain a straight, relaxed spinal column in this posture. The strength of the lift should come from your hips, and most of the weight should balance on your shoulders. To perform Bridge Pose with Long Holds:

- Lie flat on your back, relax your spine into the floor, and center your concentration to prepare for the posture.

- Bend your knees and place your feet flat on the ground, pulling your heels into your buttocks. Keep your knees and thighs parallel and slightly parted.

- Place your arms along your sides, pressing firmly into the ground with your palms facing down.

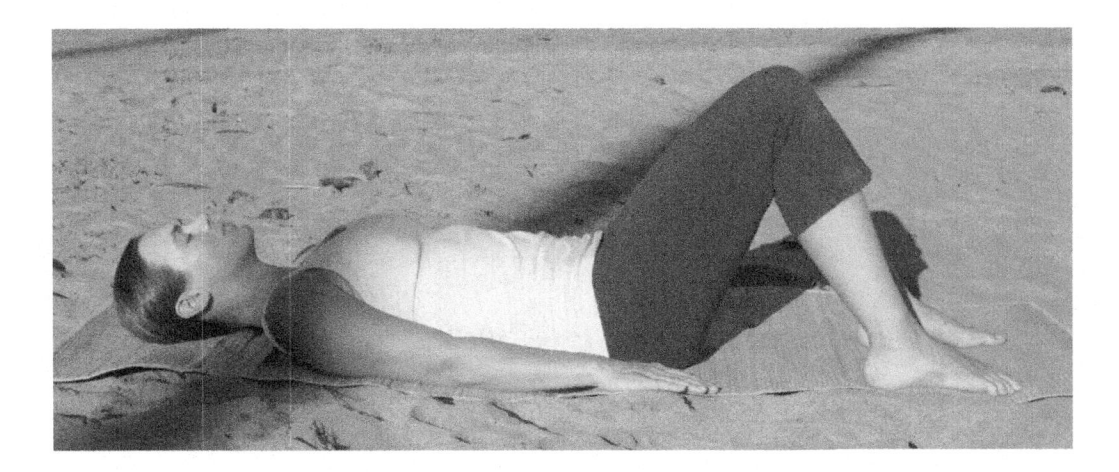

- Slowly, starting from your tailbone, lift your buttocks and back from the floor, lifting one vertebra at a time.

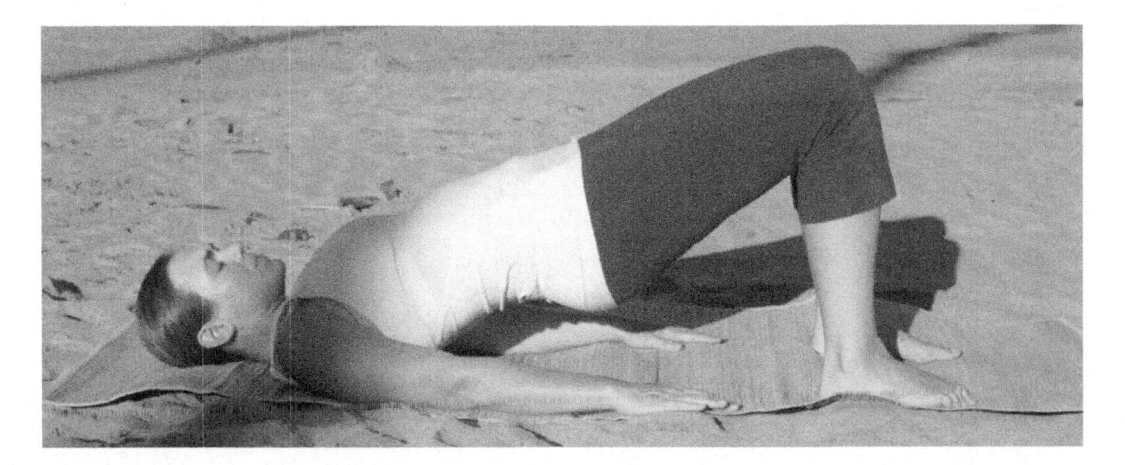

- Do not turn your head. Do not rest weight on your neck. Support yourself through the strength of your feet, arms, and shoulders.

- If flexibility allows, roll your shoulders under further. Slide your arms under your body, bringing your hands together underneath your back and clasping together your fingers and palms.

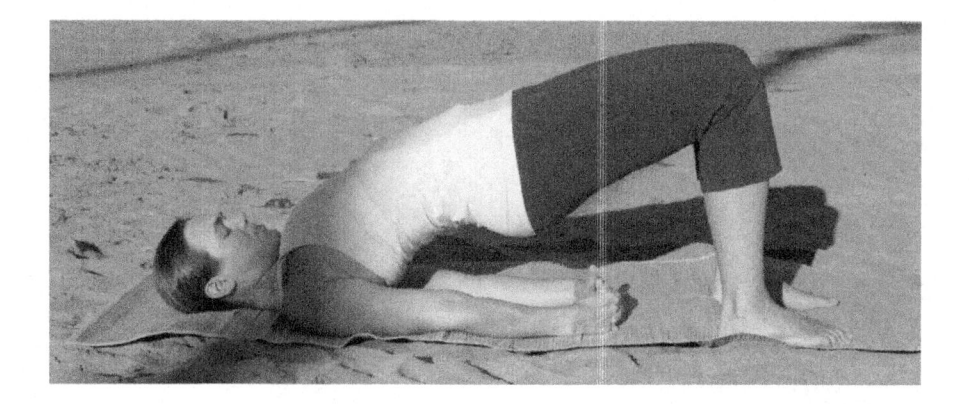

- Continue to lift up through the hips.

- Hold Bridge, performing ten Long Holds while breathing naturally.

- Release the hands to the sides.

- Slowly roll out of Bridge Pose—one vertebrae at a time—rolling the spine gently down onto the floor.

- Release your legs, relax your arms, and resume normal breathing.

Advanced Poses

The more advanced poses require more advanced yoga ability and are not necessary for pelvic rehabilitation. However, if you are capable of performing full backbends and inversions, you will see a great improvement in pelvic strength by integrating your pelvic floor exercises with these advanced yoga postures. It is very difficult to maintain a pelvic lift while using other muscles of the body. The muscles of the legs, buttocks, and abdomen are much larger muscles than those of the pelvic floor. Movement in those larger muscles takes your focus away from the pelvic region, causing you to "drop" and lose control. Learning to control your pelvic muscles while using other parts of your body will bring ultimate control over your pelvic health.

Positions like Wide-Leg Sitting Forward Bend and Happy Baby Pose are difficult postures for pelvic floor work because of the wide opening of the pelvic region. When the legs are spread wide apart, the groin and pelvis open outward. During this expansion of the entire pelvic region, it is difficult to simultaneously contract and draw in the muscles isolated within the figure eight.

For advanced postures, work each different pelvic floor technique in each different yoga pose. Try sets of ten repetitions of pelvic floor exercise per pose, discovering which poses produce the most results for your body. If a particular pose is most difficult, it is likely dealing with the weakest muscles of your pelvic floor, and therefore is the exercise you most need. However, if the advanced poses are difficult in and of themselves, do not strain yourself. Return to the moderate or beginning poses. Then work slowly on the advanced yoga poses, achieving a level of comfort within each pose before you begin pelvic exercise integration.

(1) Wide-Leg Sitting Forward Bend

Wide-Leg Sitting Forward Bend is beneficial for the strength and flexibility of the thighs, buttocks, and hips. It strengthens and encourages flexibility of the lower back, releasing tension and pressure on the nerves. Wide-Leg Sitting Forward Bend is beneficial for prevention of incontinence, menstrual cramps, and lower backache. It also encourages digestion and is a remedy for constipation. To do this pose:

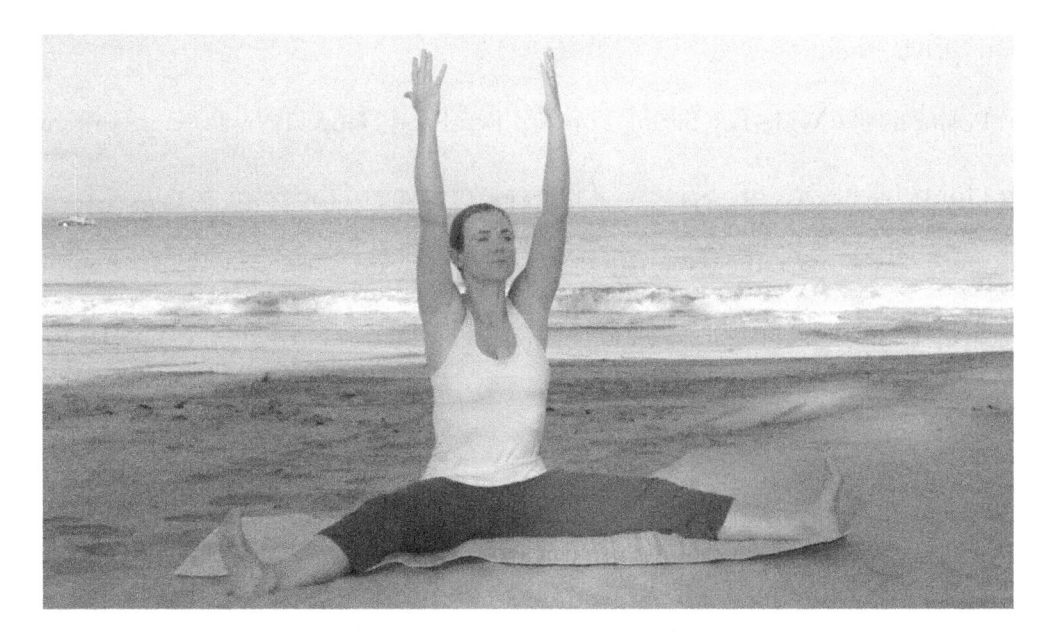

- Sit on the floor, spreading your legs apart as far as possible while still feeling comfortable. Do not strain your muscles; do not risk injury.

- Your sit bones should be firmly grounded into the floor with your spine lifting and fluid and the crown of your head reaching toward the ceiling.

- Flex your feet, pulling your toes toward you with your heels pulling away from your body. The arch of your foot should be stretched out and slightly lifted. Keep your knees rotated up toward the ceiling. Do not let your knees fall in. Inward falling knees are a natural tendency in this pose, but they can be damaging to your knees.

- While inhaling, stretch your arms over your head. Lift your rib cage, look up, and lift your chin. Keep your shoulders down, away from your ears.

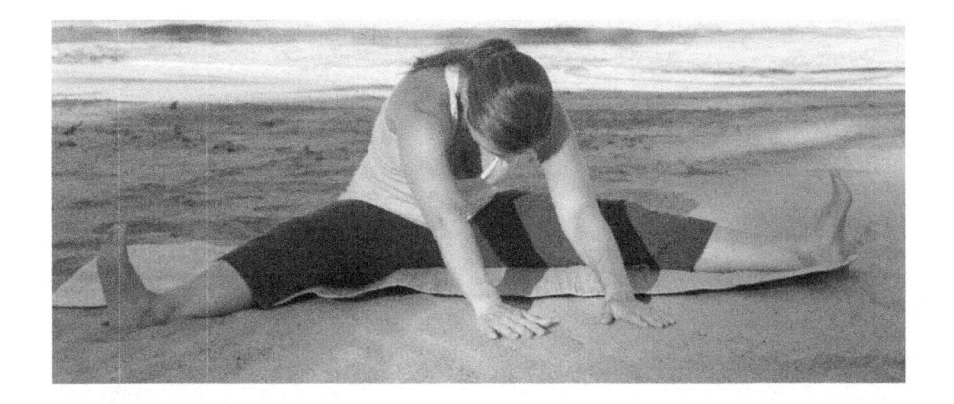

- While exhaling, bend forward from your hips, not from your waist. Keep your torso long, reaching your hands along the floor between your legs. Stretch long. Rather than trying to put your head on the floor, attempt to reach your chest to the floor. Pull it forward with your hands, maintaining proper forms for your knees (up toward the ceiling) and toes (flexed).

- Hold. Breathe gently and naturally, while performing ten pelvic floor contractions.

- Relax and release. Bring your hands to your waist.

- Inhale, lifting your chest with a flat, comfortable back. Then return to center.

- Use your hands on the outside of each thigh to push your legs together.

- Rest your legs before getting up.

(2) Happy Baby Pose

Happy Baby Pose stretches the inner thighs, pelvis, and hamstrings. Because it is a posture that puts you into a "baby" position, it can leave you feeling emotionally vulnerable. Happy Baby can also help you to feel happy and light. To perform this pose:

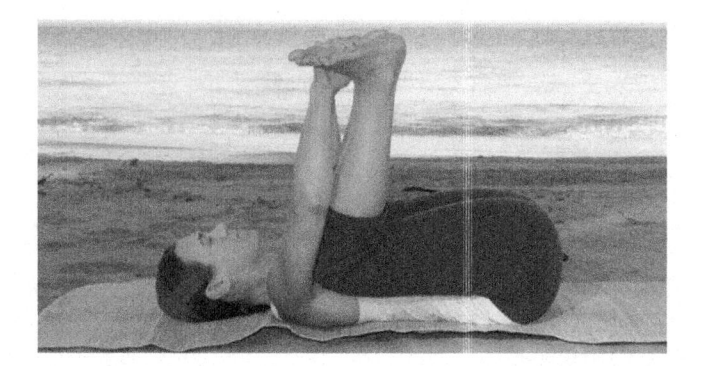

- Lie flat on your back.

- Bring your knees into your chest.

- Pull your knees out to the sides of your body and lift your feet toward the ceiling.

- Reach inside your legs and place your hands inside the arches of your feet (right hand in your right arch, left hand in left arch.)

- Use your hands to stretch your legs, opening your hips and pulling your knees down and out toward your armpits.

- Your tailbone will naturally round and lift off the floor; however, work to pull your lower back toward the floor, grounding with each breath.

- Hold this stretch, relaxing and breathing comfortably.

- Perform ten pelvic floor exercises.

- Relax. Then release your hands from your feet.

- Breathe and relax.

- Release your legs.

- Rest and then roll onto one side.

- Use the strength of your hands to push up gently from the floor into Simple Sitting.

(3) Downward Facing Dog Pose

Tight hamstrings can pull on the pelvis and alter the natural tilt of the pelvic bowl. This can cause backaches and pelvic disorders, and make the legs tired due to improper balance and posture. Downward Dog is a wonderful posture because it inverts the body in a gentle way, without pressure on the spine, thus providing the benefits of inversion without the difficulties and potential injury risk of advanced inversions such as Headstand and Shoulderstand. Downward Dog is also excellent because it relaxes hamstrings and stretches the muscles of the buttocks and lower back. Downward Dog also lengthens the spine and loosens the neck, releasing the spine from the weight of the head, allowing the upper vertebrae to relax. To perform Downward Dog:

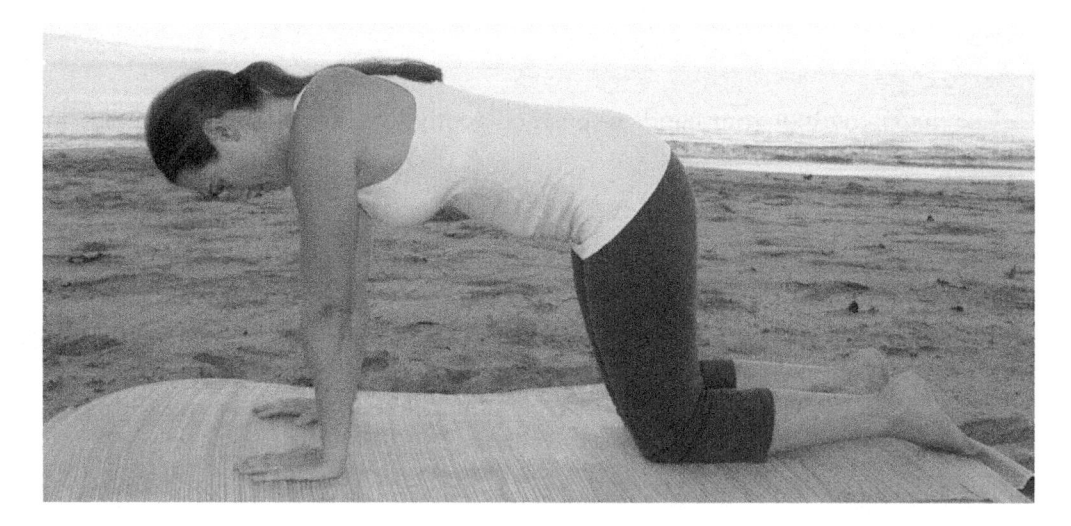

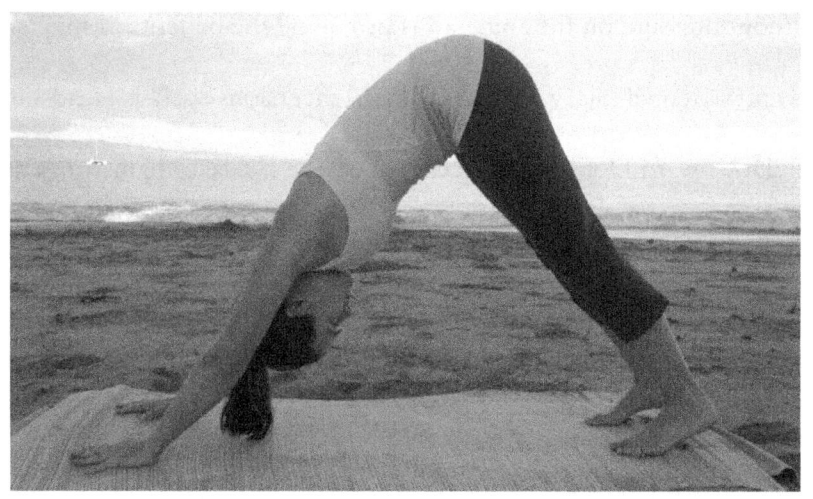

- Start on your hands and knees with your hands straight below your shoulders and your knees straight below your hipbones (See Cat-Cow for details).

- Press your palms firmly into the ground, flattening your entire palm.

- With your knees bent, begin to lift your hips toward the ceiling, tilting your pelvis back.

- Slowly begin to straighten your legs, moving your heels toward the floor.

- Push your hands firmly into the mat. Take the weight off your shoulders, and pull your shoulder blades together. At the same time expand and open your chest, pushing the stability of the pose back toward your heels.

- Breathe deeply, relaxing your neck and letting gravity stretch out the weight of your head.

- With each breath, feel your body weight shift more toward your heels. As you stretch your legs, reach your heels to the floor, and then release your shoulders.

- In Downward Dog, perform ten pelvic floor contractions.

- To release, bend your knees gently, and return to your starting position.

- Relax the tops of your feet onto the ground, sit back on your heels, relax your chest against your thighs, and rest in Child's Pose.

(4) Fish Pose

Fish Pose helps the neck and spine to loosen and open. This pose expands the ribcage and opens the lungs as well. To perform the Fish Pose:

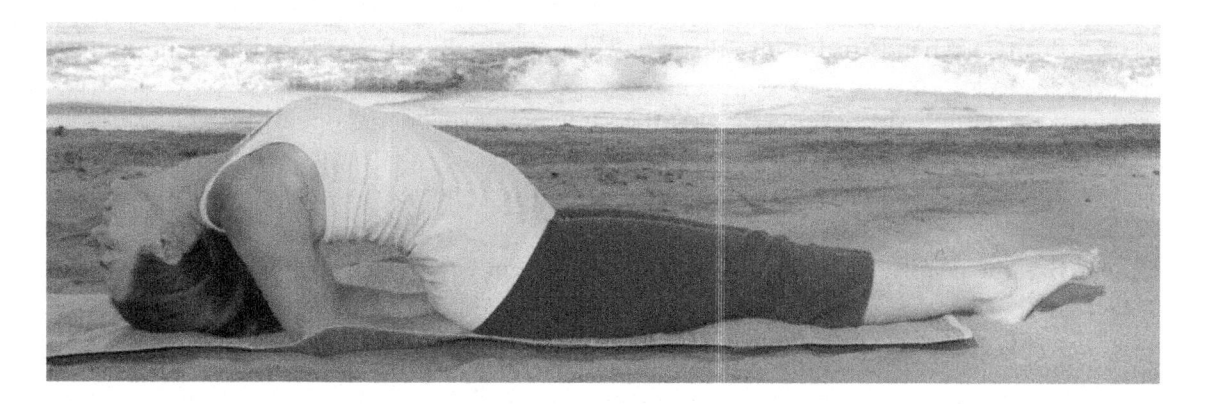

- Lie down on your back, and place your hands under your hips (left hand under left hip, right hand under right hip).

- Pull your elbows under your body, propping yourself and lifting your chest.

- Arch your neck back and lift your chin to the ceiling, moving the crown of your head back to the floor behind you. Lift your pelvic floor, and hold for a ten-count long hold.

- Feel how your neck relaxes and opens. Breathe naturally.

- Release. Then return your neck to a normal position and relax the pelvic floor. Release your hands from under your hips. Then lie down, relaxed and calm.

(5) Backbend (Wheel)

The Backbend, or Wheel, is one of the most difficult of yoga postures. It requires patience, diligent effort, a calm mind, and strength of the entire body. Wheel encourages both strength and flexibility of the hips, chest, back, arms, legs, and neck; in fact, it works the entire body. Wheel stimulates every chakra, filling the body with energy. Because Wheel requires so much strength, energy, and flexibility, you will know you have achieved true control of your pelvic muscles if you can practice your pelvic floor exercises while maintaining the Wheel Pose. To do the Wheel:

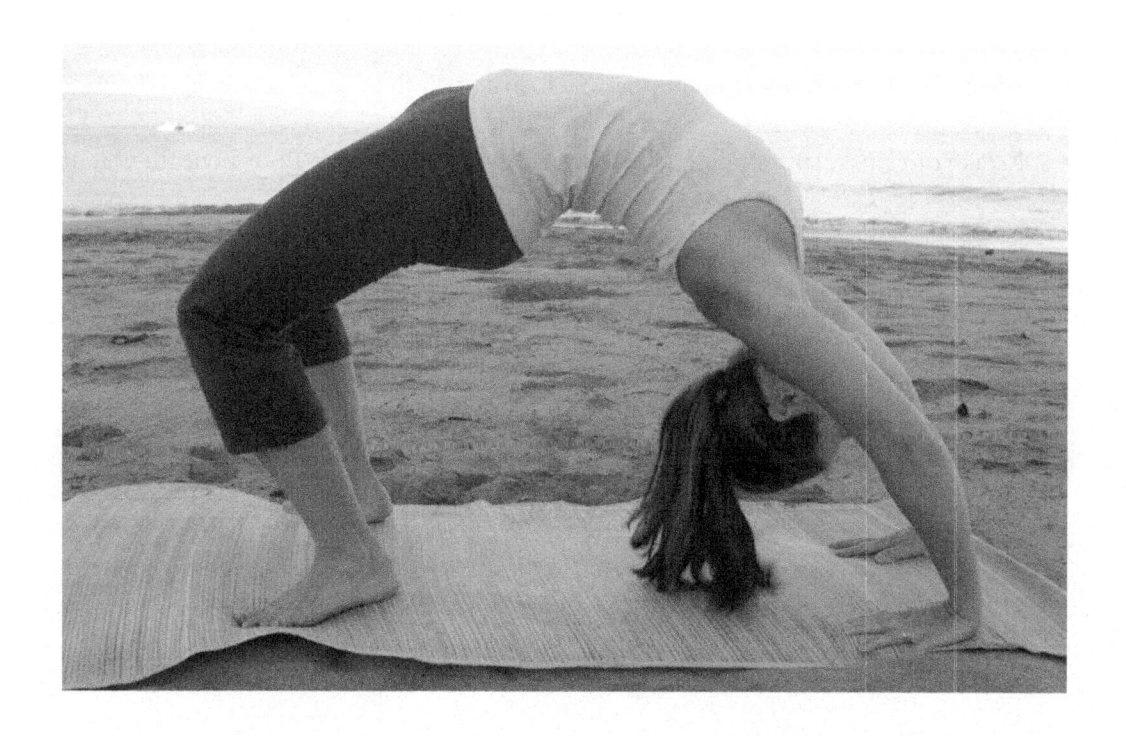

- Lie flat on your back.

- Bend your knees, placing your feet flat on the floor and drawing your heels toward your buttocks. Your legs should be parallel, drawing straight out of your hipbones.

- Lift your arms over your head and bend your elbows. Bring your hands underneath so that your fingers point toward your shoulders. Keep your arms close to your head.

- Start at the bottom, and use the strength of your thighs and pelvis to begin to lift your body into the air. Inhale as you perform this part of the pose.

- Use your abdominals and back, and lift the pose higher.

- Then use your shoulders and upper back, lifting all the way into Wheel.

- Relax your neck, stretching backwards slightly to look at the floor beneath you, if possible. Make sure not to strain.

- If you are comfortable and secure in Wheel, slowly walk your feet in toward your hands, tightening the circle of your backbend.

- Lift and curve through the entire spine. Be careful of "pseudo-backbends," where only one portion of the back lifts and the rest remains stuck in a tight, straight position.

- Breathe deeply and rhythmically, holding the backbend without strain or force. If it becomes uncomfortable, release onto the floor.

- Hold Wheel and breathe, performing ten pelvic floor exercises. Begin with Quick-Flicks, progressing to more difficult techniques as you build greater strength and stamina.

- Exhale, releasing your body slowly to the floor. Starting with the upper body, and then roll the spine down slowly and calmly.

- Curl your knees into your chest and tuck your forehead into your knees, counter-posing the stretch to relax.

- Release onto the floor and relax in Corpse position.

Supportive Yoga Exercises

True Pelvic Yoga health requires more than yoga exercise focusing on the pelvic region. The body is composed of many parts, which comprise a single unit. In addition to your Pelvic Yoga practice, you must make time for Pelvic Yoga support. At least three times per week, exercise those parts of your body that support your reproductive organs—your abdominal muscles; your thighs, pelvis, and buttocks; and your back. You should also engage in aerobic activity to exercise your heart and lungs.

Yoga's deep breathing regulated with stretching and strengthening the muscles is an ideal method of encouraging health and fitness. The Pelvic Yoga support exercises will encourage your Pelvic Yoga work, but they will also benefit your appearance and ability to participate in life and physical activity.

Supportive Exercises for Abdominal Strengthening

(1) Stomach Contractions / Abdominal Lift

This exercise is "Uddyiana Bandha" in Sanskrit. Like Mulabandha, Uddyiana Bandha is a yogic lock intended to channel energy up the spine to increase spiritual and psychic powers. Physiologically, it stimulates and tones the entire abdominal region, encouraging health of the urinary, digestive, and reproductive systems. It strengthens the abdominal muscles and helps support the pelvic hammock. It also tones the nerves of the solar plexus and supports relaxation. To do this exercise:

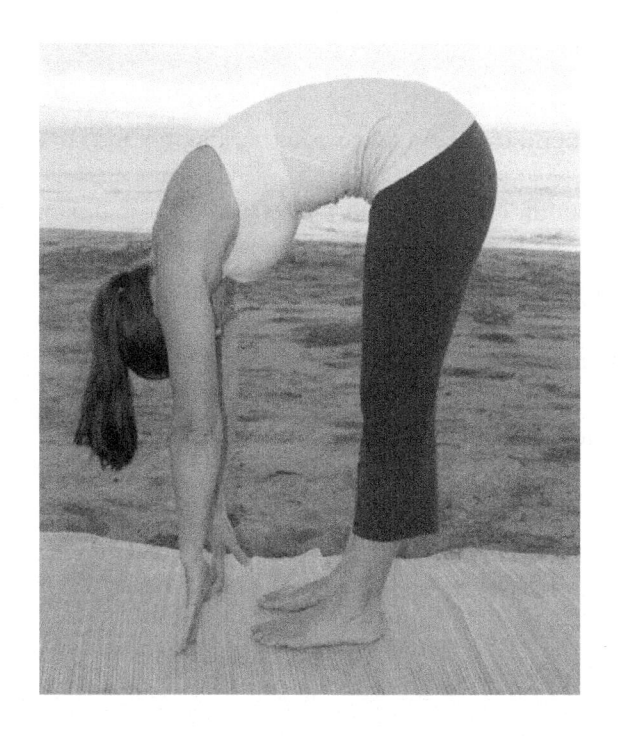

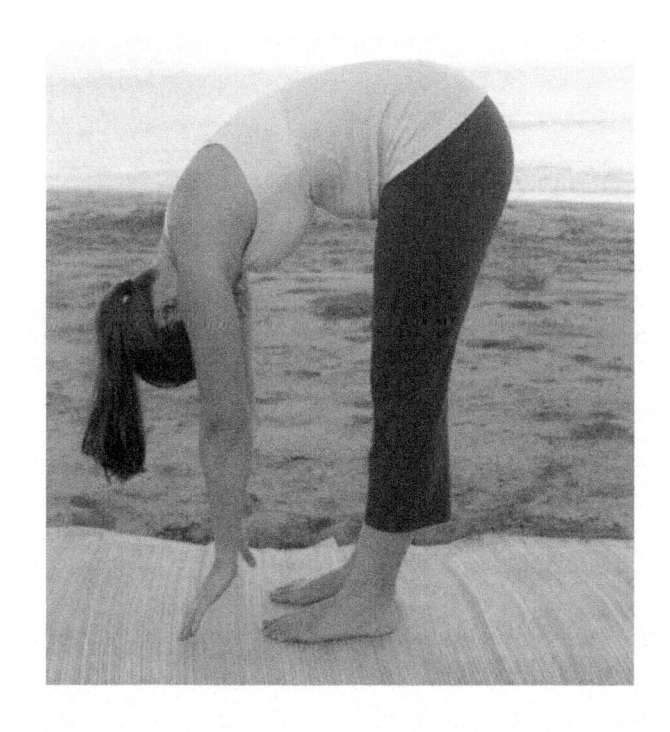

- While standing, bend over and place your hands on your knees (or your shins, ankles, or the floor, depending on flexibility). You may sit if that is more comfortable.
- Inhale completely. Raise your diaphragm and contract your abdominal muscles until everything under your ribs feels hollow.
- Exhale completely. Hold your body with no breath.
- With no breath, suck in your lower stomach (only your lower stomach) as if you are absorbing your pelvis, abdomen, and belly button back into your spine. Hold.
- Release. Breathe normally.
- Repeat.
- Relax. Breathe in and out gently, returning to natural, uncontrolled breath.

Advanced practice, based on Kundalini technique:

- While standing, bend over and place your hands on your knees (or your shins, ankles, or the floor, depending on flexibility). You may sit if that is more comfortable.
- Inhale completely.
- Then exhale completely. Hold your body with no breath.
- With no breath, suck in your lower stomach—only your lower stomach—as if you are absorbing your pelvis, abdomen, and belly button back into your spine.

- Pump your stomach back and forth with no breath. At the same time, bring your abdomen back to your spine—releasing, pulling it in, and then releasing again. Repeat this several times.

- Release. Breathe normally.

- Repeat.

- Relax. Breathe in and out gently, returning to natural, uncontrolled breath.

(2) Kundalini Sitting Twists

This is a wonderful energizing exercise. Two minutes of this in the morning will awaken your spine and charge your whole day. It is also good for stimulating the digestive system, toning the abdominal muscles, and bringing greater flexibility to the spine and waist. To perform the Sitting Twists:

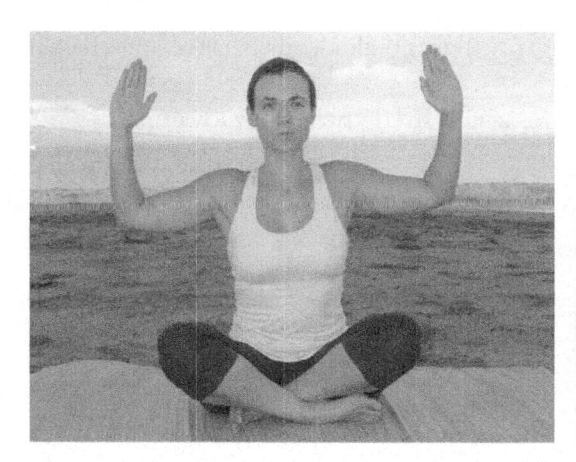

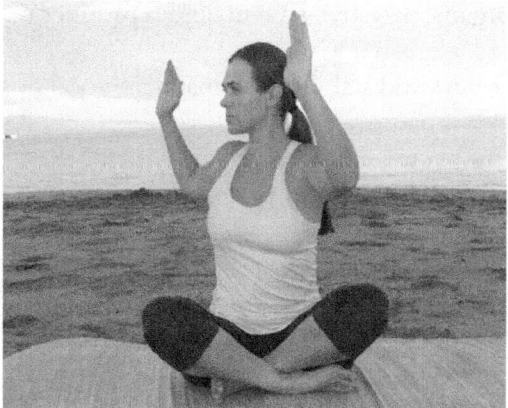

- Sit in a comfortable, cross-legged position.

- Lift your arms straight out of your shoulders. Bend them at your elbows with your fingers pointing to the sky and your palms facing forward. This is a goalpost position, and it is great for expanding your chest.

- Close your eyes and take your energy within.

- Twist your body from side to side, moving from the waist. Feel your spine warming, your waist being worked, and your internal organs toning. Feel the energy channeling up your spine. Allow your head to move gently with you as you twist, keeping your neck in line with the spine.

(3) Angle Balance and Wide-Leg Angle Balance

This exercise is an excellent abdominal strengthener. It builds support for internal organs, digestive system, and reproductive organs. It also builds your balance and challenges you to find stability and maintain good posture, which strengthens your lower back. To do this pose:

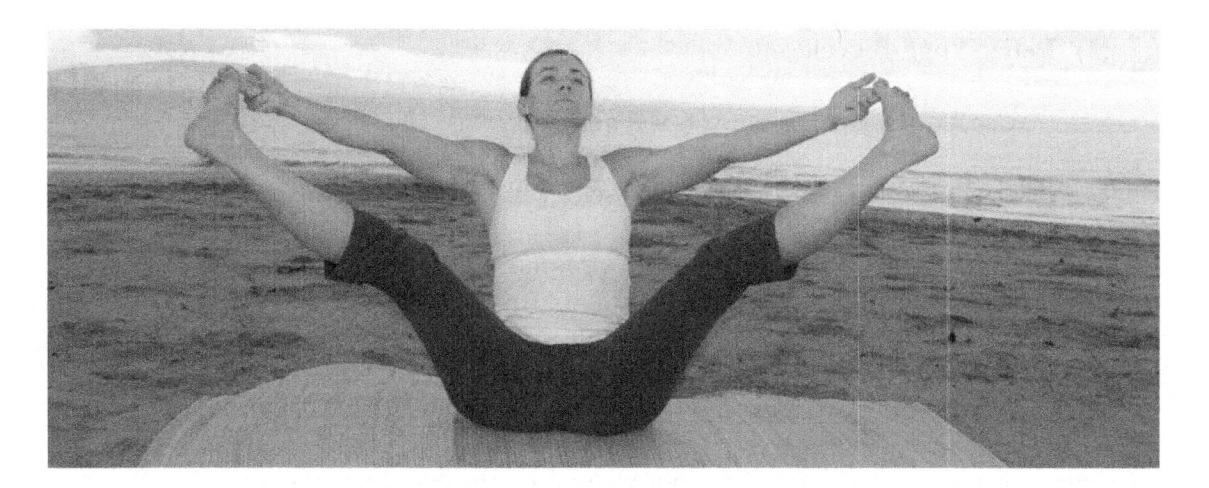

- While sitting on the ground, center your weight on your sit bones.

- Bend your knees into your chest, but keep your chest lifted and your back straight.

- Take your big toes with the index and middle fingers of each hand.

- Pull your shoulders back as you pull the chest forward, straightening your legs and balancing on your bottom. Keep your chest lifted to keep your spine straight. Do not slouch and lift through the legs.

- The focal point in these exercises is the big toes.

This additional level also stretches and strengthens the legs. It also requires a deeper level of concentration to balance and maintain stability.

- If you are flexible enough and would like to take the pose farther, open your legs to your sides while carefully maintaining your balance. At the same time, maintain your grip on your big toes. Keep your legs straight, if possible.

(4) Pelvic Yoga Bicycle

Usually, weak pelvic muscles will not work while you are using other muscles. Yoga Bicycle teaches you to use your pelvic muscles while using other muscles simultaneously. The Yoga Bicycle improves digestion and prevents constipation. It tones the abdominal muscles and challenges your concentration. It is important to keep the movement synchronized with your breath. Do not let yourself automatically fall into a quick motion without breathing. In addition, it is normal to drop the pelvic floor repeatedly in this exercise. If this happens, pick it up again and continue. As your strength improves, you will get achieve the desired results. To do the Yoga Bicycle:

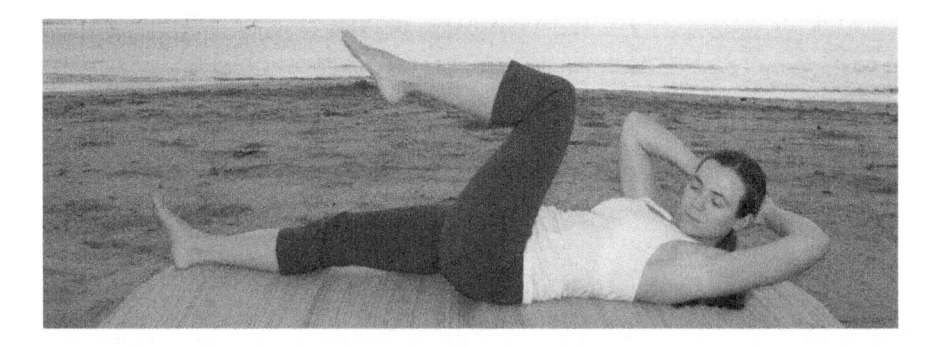

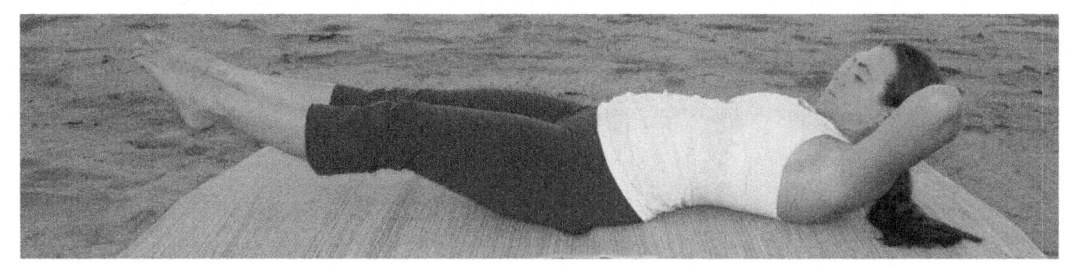

- Lie flat on your back, comfortable and relaxed.

- Using the Elevator technique, lift your pelvic muscles to the second floor.

- Contract your abdominal muscles.

- Slowly lift your right elbow and left knee to one another, while tucking in your chin and exhaling as you lift.

- Inhale, releasing to the ground. Continue holding your pelvic muscles on the second floor as you release.

- Slowly lift your left elbow and right knee to one another, while tucking in your chin and exhaling as you lift.

- Inhale, releasing to the ground. Continue holding your pelvic muscles on the second floor as you release.

- As you get stronger, learn to hold your feet and upper body gently lifted from the floor throughout the set. This will build even more abdominal strength.

Try to repeat for ten full sets (ten per side, for a total of twenty) WITHOUT ever releasing the pelvic muscles. This is a VERY long hold. At first, you will only be able to do one or two without losing the pelvic contraction. Gradually build pelvic strength.

(5) Reclined Cobbler's Pose Crunches

Cobbler's Pose both stretches and strengthens the legs and low back. Reclined crunches in Cobbler's Pose should be performed with care, so that you do not injure your back. These are very difficult but quickly build strength in the abdominals. If you cannot do Elevators, do Reclined Cobbler's Pose Crunches with Contract-Release or with Long Holds.

You can also do them without pelvic floor exercises, in order to focus more energy on the abdominals. To perform these crunches:

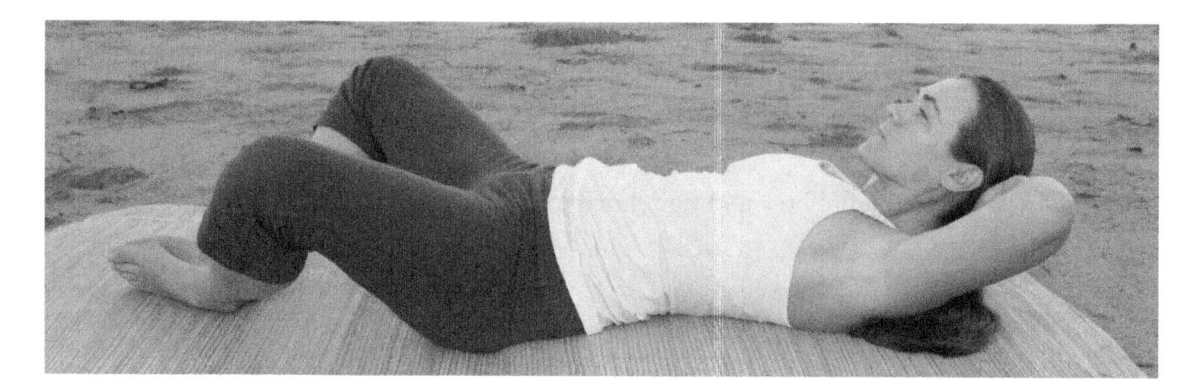

- Sit on the floor with a straight back. Bring the soles of your feet together, pulling your heels toward your thighs.

- While breathing deeply, hold your toes. Maintain a straight back, feel the outward rotation of your thigh muscles, and concentrate on the opening of your groin.

- If you are comfortable, stay in Cobbler's Pose. If you would like to try a deeper opening, gently relax back onto your elbows.

- While keeping your feet together and pulled in toward the groin, release onto your back. Relax your arms and rest your back fully along the ground. Concentrate to feel the full length of your spine.

- If you experience discomfort in your legs and hips, place a blanket or a pillow underneath each knee for support. Be sure to keep your thighs open but use enough support to prevent muscle strain.

- Cross your arms gently over your chest.

- Lift your pelvic floor muscles to the second level.

- Holding your pelvic muscles, curl your chin into your chest. Lift your shoulders off the floor to do an abdominal crunch.

- Hold the crunch for one to two seconds, and then release your back gently to the floor.

- Repeat up to fifty times, holding your pelvic muscles at the second floor throughout. If you drop the second floor, relax, contract again, and continue with the crunches. Your goal is to gain the muscular control to hold the second floor contraction throughout the duration of fifty crunches.

(6) Boat Pose

There are several poses called Boat in the various yoga traditions. This pose is Navasana, from the Ashtanga practice series. It is similar to Angle Balance and Wide-Angle Balance Pose. It is a great abdominal strengthener. It also strengthens the mid-back, if done correctly. The important thing is not to hunch your back. Instead, keep yourself lifting forward through the chest.

The pose progresses through several stages. Stay at the stage that is comfortable for you, challenging your abilities but respecting your body's needs and limitations. Yoga is a personal practice, above all things, and we always need to remember that sense of self-respect. It is better to be at a lower stage with integrity, and hold it for a long count of five or ten deep breaths, than to pop into and fall out of a more difficult stage. Yoga poses bring benefits when held through deep breaths with integrity. It is about quality, not quantity or level of difficulty. To do this pose:

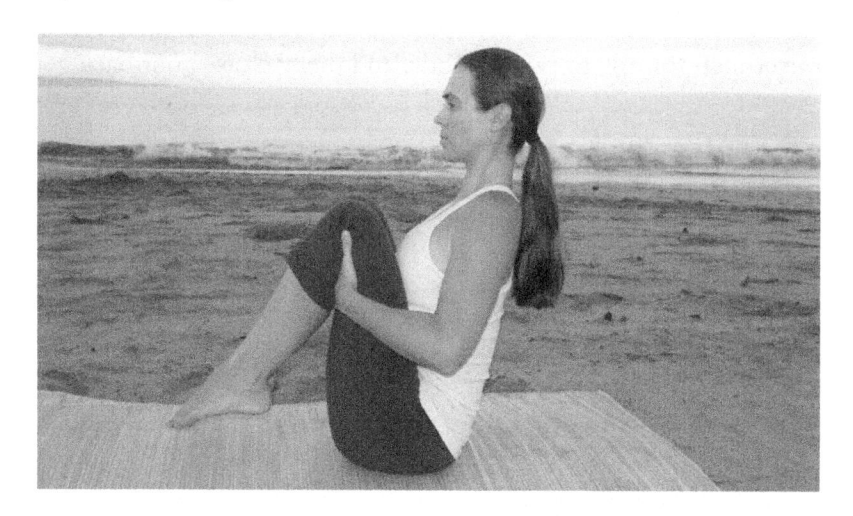

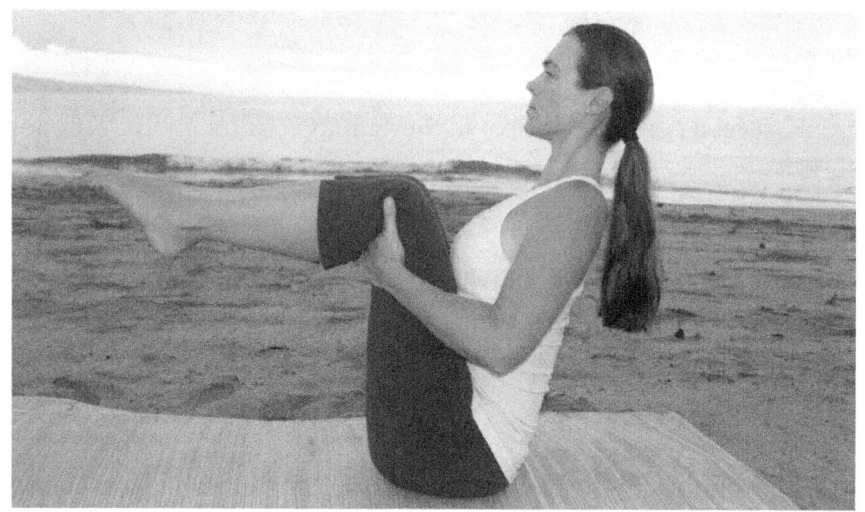

- Sitting on the ground, center your weight on your sit bones.
- Bend your knees into your chest, keeping your chest lifted and your back straight.

- Stage one: Hold your legs just behind the knees. Lift your shins so that they are parallel with the floor. Point your toes away from you. Maintain this pose, balance, and breathe.

- Stage 2: Continue to hold the position of your legs. Release your hands from behind your legs. Stretch your arms along each side of your legs with your palms facing in and your fingers extending away from you. Keep your chest lifted and your spine straight and strong as you balance. Breathe deeply, feeling the energy extend through your fingertips.

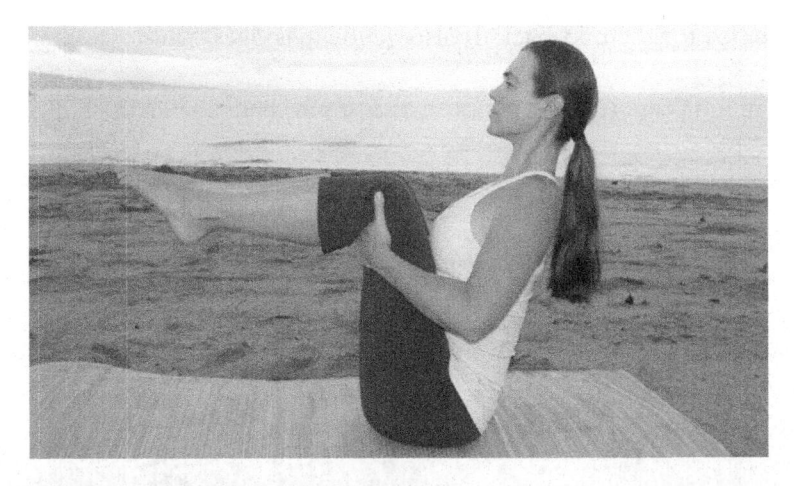

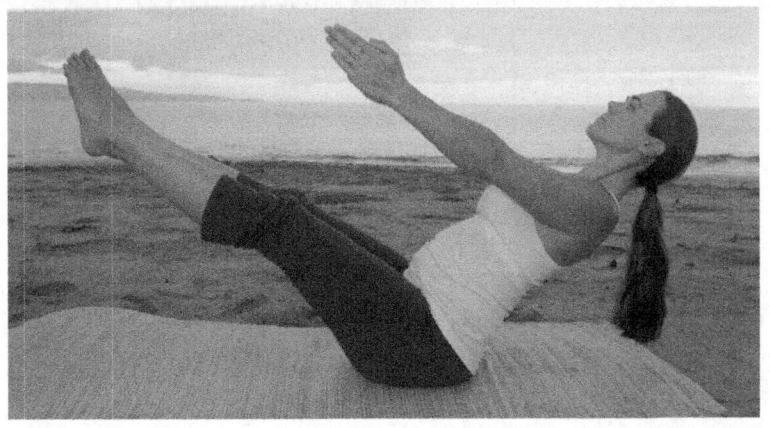

- Stage 3: Without letting your posture sink, slowly begin to straighten your legs. Keep lifting through the chest. Bring your body into a nice angled posture with your bottom resting on the ground. At the same time, extend out and up through your head and feet. Extend through your fingertips toward your toes. Your big toes are the focal point. Breathe deeply.

(7) Airplane

Airplane strengthens your back and stretches your abdominal muscles. It is a wonderful exercise for the mid-back. It also gently massages your lower belly, giving your digestive system a nice workout. This pose also strengthens the arms. This is the pose sometimes called Boat in other yoga traditions. To perform the Airplane:

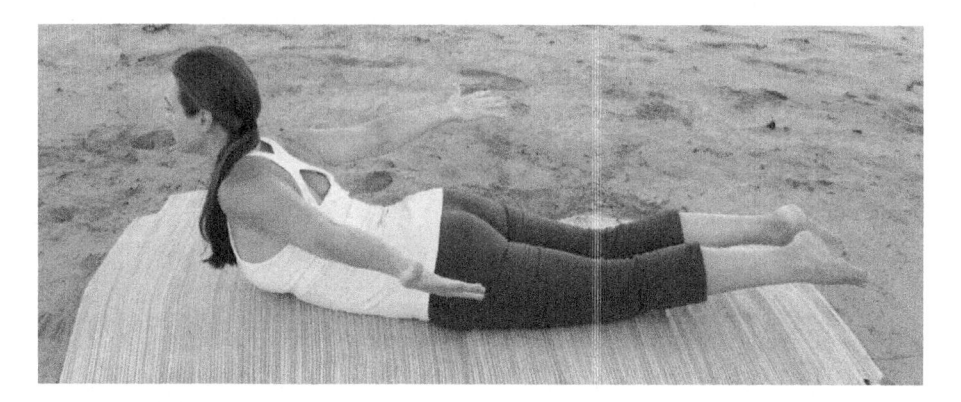

- Lie on your belly.

- Stretch your arms above your head with your palms facing each other.

- Rest on your chin, softly gazing forward.

- Gently squeeze your legs and toes together.

- While inhaling, lift up through the chest and the legs, lifting the arms and legs off the ground. Your belly should be relaxed into the ground as you gently lift your cheat and extend your arms and legs. Keep your limbs straight.

- Breathe into this pose, feeling your body rise and fall with your breath.

- When you are comfortable with the next stage, open your arms to your sides, straight from the shoulders. Face your palms downward as you lift through the arms to stretch your chest and strengthen your mid-back. Continue to lift through the legs, feeling your body rise and fall with your breath. Your belly gets a good deep stretch and massage as you maintain this pose.

(8) Locust

Locust is similar to Airplane. It is, likewise, a good stretch and massage for the belly and digestive organs and a great strengthener for the back, specifically the lower back. Locust tones and strengthens the lower back, buttocks, and backs of thighs. To do the Locust Pose:

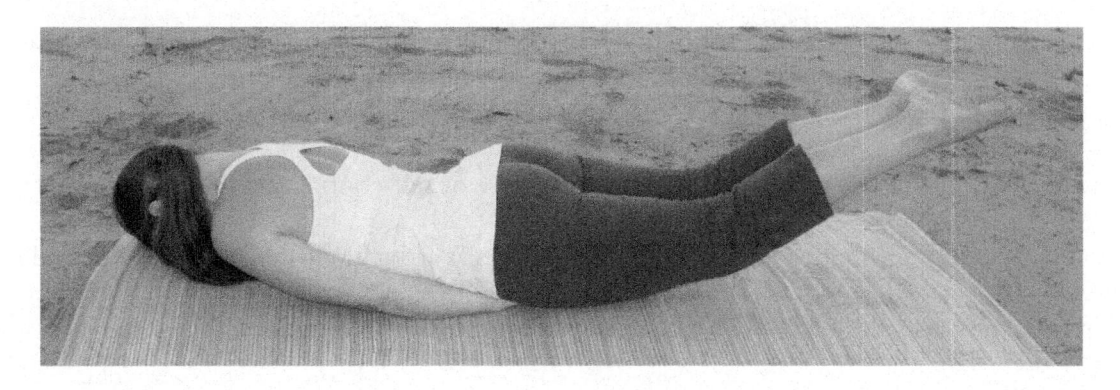

- Lie on your belly.

- Make your hands into soft fists. Place your fists under your body, approximately under your lower belly or upper groin area.

- Rest gently on your forehead.

- Squeeze your legs together gently from the tips of your toes to the top of your upper thighs.

- Inhale. Keeping your forehead grounded on the yoga mat and your chest relaxed onto the floor, lift up through the legs.

- Keep your legs straight if possible, stretching through your toes and feeling the lower back and buttocks strengthening in the effort.

- Breathe as you hold the pose.

Supportive Exercises for the Thighs, Pelvis, and Buttocks

(1)   Warrior One

Warrior One revitalizes the entire body. It strengthens the legs and buttocks, builds heat in the core of the body, and energizes the upper body. When held through several deep breaths, Warrior brings endurance and a greater sense of self-confidence. It can tone your body while helping you to achieve emotional courage. Warrior elongates the spine, opens the hip area, improves flexibility of the torso, and strengthens the feet, ankles, knees, and legs. To do Warrior One:

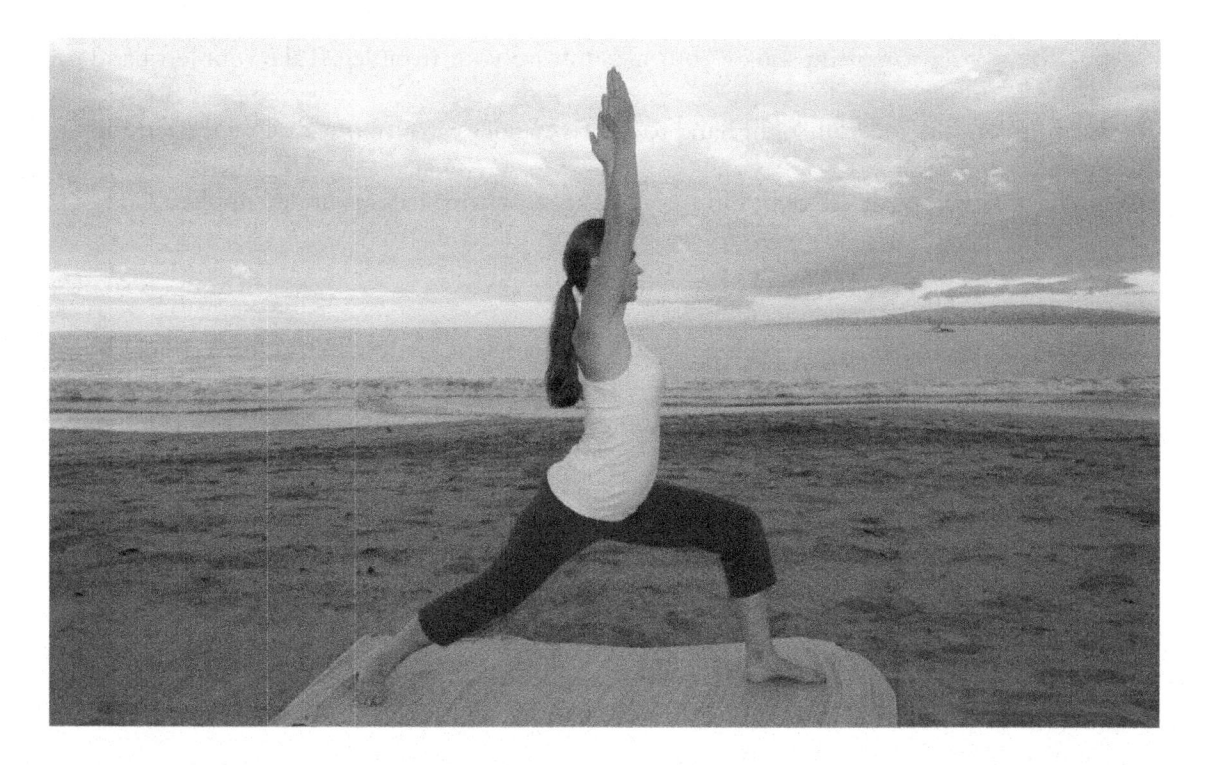

- Begin standing in Mountain Pose. Center your energy in the core of your body. Lift your toes gently to center your balance on the arches of the feet, evenly distributing the weight between the balls and the heels of the feet.

- Step your feet about three to four feet apart. Correct distancing will place your ankles directly under your wrists when your arms are out-stretched.

- To begin with left-side Warrior One, turn your left foot out and angle your right foot in slightly.

- Rotate your torso and square your hips toward your front leg. Take your left hand to your left hip and your right hand to the right side of your bottom. Pull the left hip back as you push the right hip forward, keeping your feet grounded in place, and thus squaring your pelvis to face forward.

- Bend into the left knee, taking it into a right angle if you can. Your knee should be directly over the ankle; do not extend the knee past the ankle because this can injure the knee joint. Using the strength of your inner thigh, pull your left knee toward the little toe side of your foot; this protects your knee as well.

- Find your balance and stability in the pose. Keep your upper body squared over the hips. Do not lean forward over the front leg. Hands begin at the waist.

- If you feel strong and comfortable, lift your arms while inhaling and stretch long through your ribs. Keep your shoulders down and away from your ears as you lift through the fingertips. At the same time, ground down through your feet, lengthening your spine and body. If you feel comfortable doing so, lift your chin gently to look at your fingertips.

- Breathe. Holding the pose for five to ten deep breaths.

- Repeat on the opposite side.

(2) Crescent Pose

Crescent Pose builds on Warrior One, adding the element of a gentle backbend. The crescent is the symbol of yoga, so this pose can have significant symbolic power. This pose expands the chest and strengthens the back. The weight is balanced mostly on the back leg, to allow you to relax into the backbend. With each exhalation, you can feel yourself stretching farther back. To complete the Crescent Pose:

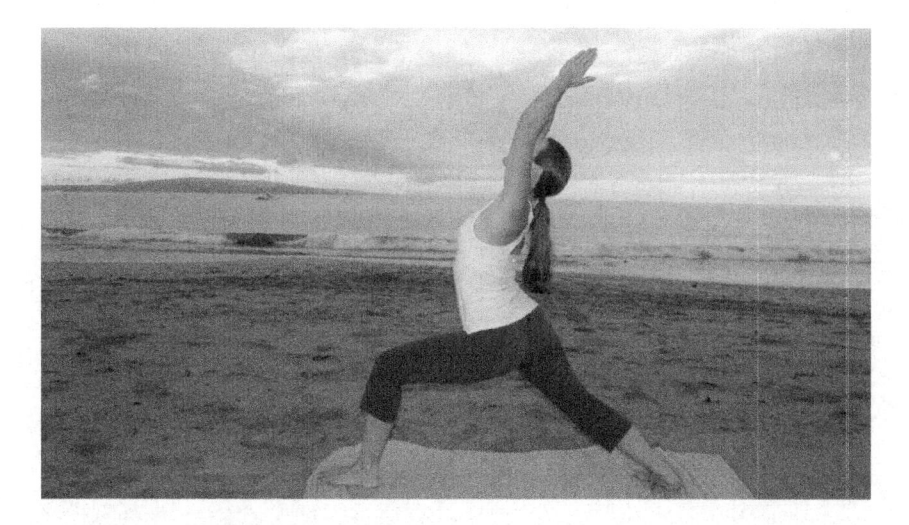

- Begin in Warrior One, with your arms extended over your head.

- Bring your palms to touch.

- Arch back gently, stretching through your fingertips as you lift up your chest and move your head comfortably back.

- As you move into a backbend, keep your lower back, legs, and buttocks strong. Be careful not to end up with an exaggerated swayback.

- Breathe. Hold the pose for five to ten deep breaths.

- Repeat on the opposite side.

(3) Warrior Two

Warrior Two is a great thigh strengthener. It also develops the core of the body, just as Warrior One does. Warrior Two is an important pose in weight loss and weight maintenance. To do this pose:

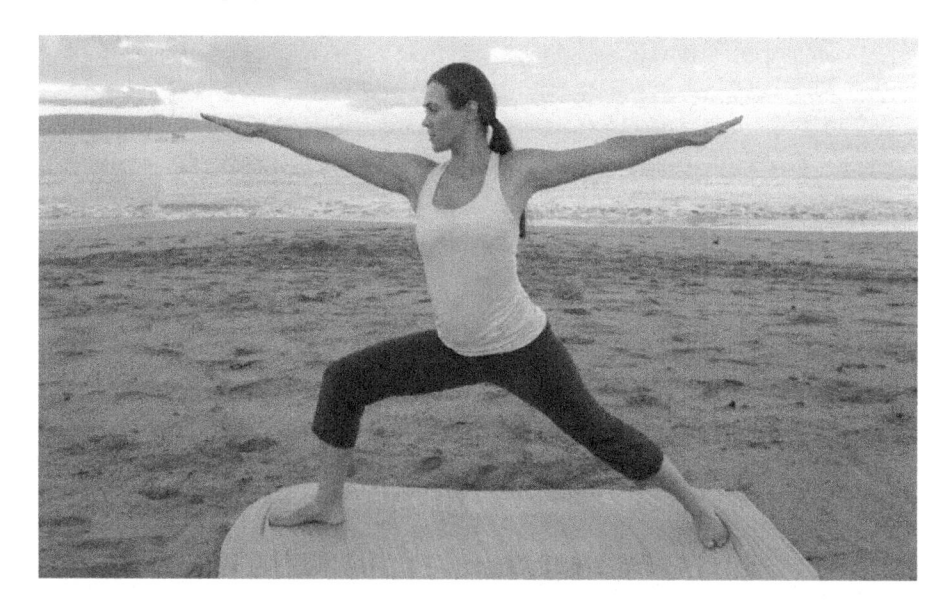

- Begin standing in Mountain Pose. Center your energy in the core of your body. Lift your toes gently to center your balance on the arches of your feet, evenly distributing the weight between the balls and the heels of your feet.

- Spread your feet about three or four feet apart, so that your ankles are directly underneath the wrists when your arms are outstretched.

- Begin with right side Warrior Two: turn your right toes out and your left toes in slightly. Place your left hand on your left hip and your right hand on your right buttock. Pull your left hip back as you push your right buttock forward. Use the strengths of your legs to help with this motion. Rotate your left thigh outward and right thigh inward, working to bring your pelvis into a flat plane. (Imagine your body is in between two walls, and your pelvis has to be parallel between those walls.)

- While inhaling, lift your arms straight up from the shoulders. Pull long through your fingertips, moving your fingers away from you in each direction to expand your shoulders and open your chest.

- Bend into your right knee, taking your knee into a right angle if you can. Make sure that your knee is directly above the ankle to protect your knee. To work your inner thigh and protect your knee, pull your knee out toward the little toe side of the foot. Keep pulling back through your left hip and thigh to keep the pelvis as flat as possible.

- Look over the fingers of the right hand. Keep your upper body squared in the center of your legs. Do not lean over your right leg.

- Breathe. Hold the pose for five to ten deep breaths. Your face should be calm and relaxed. Do not strain.

- Repeat on the opposite side.

(4) Side-Angle Pose

By taking Warrior Two into a deeper stretch, you lengthen the side of your body and further activate your leg muscles. Work to lengthen through your fingertips, extending from the tip of the fingers down through the grounded foot for a long, lean line of your spine. To perform Side-Angle Pose:

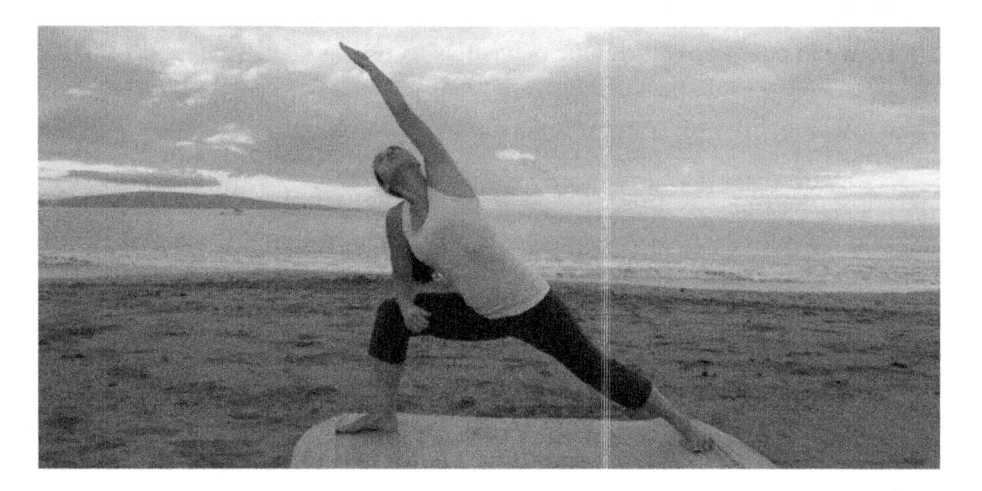

- Begin from Warrior Two.

- Take your right elbow down to your right knee, maintaining the integrity of the leg positioning.

- Inhale with your left arm in the air. Stretch along your left ear, extending your fingertips as far as you can.

- Rotate your ribs around your body. Pull your left ribs back, gently twisting your internal organs.

- Look toward the fingertips of your left hand. Feel your neck lengthen.

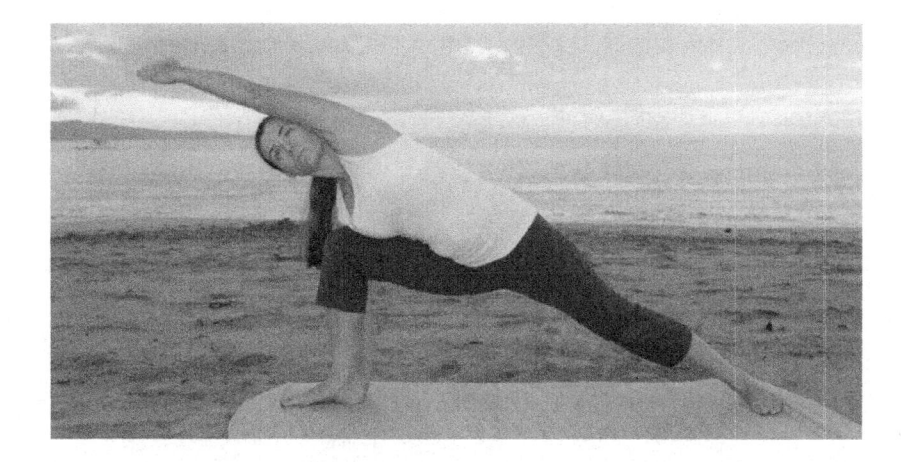

- If you have the flexibility and feel comfortable moving farther, bring your right hand down to the floor on the outside of your right foot. Push the outside of your knee gently into your arm to keep opening up the inner thigh.

- Feel your body lengthen through chest and back. Extend the fingertips of your left hand past your head. Look up.

- Find a sense of comfort in this pose. Relax into the stretch while maintaining the strength and integrity of the pose.

- Breathe. Hold for five to ten deep breaths.

- Repeat on the opposite side.

(5) Triangle

Triangle stretches the spine and spinal nerves. This pose encourages hip flexibility, leg flexibility, and body awareness. At first, it can be difficult to tell if you are correctly positioned in Triangle, and learning that sense of the placement of your body can bring powerful awareness. Triangle also helps to adjust the sacrum and lower back, improving structural alignment. To do this pose:

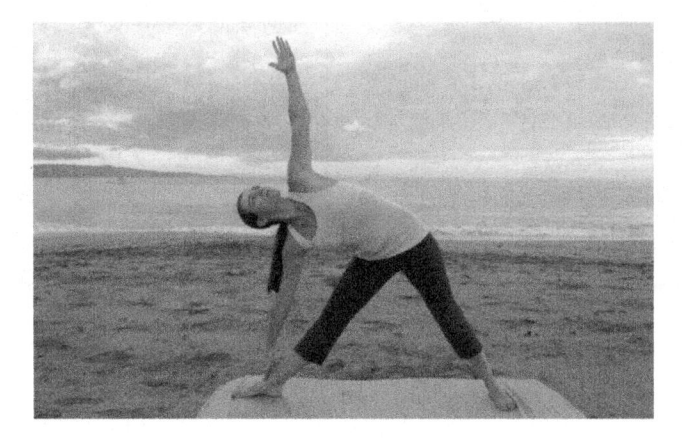

- Begin by standing in Mountain Pose.

- Spread your feet about two to three feet apart. They should be as far apart as the length of one of your legs, forming an equilateral triangle.

- Point your right toes outward in a straight line with your shin; turn your left foot in.

- Work on flattening your pelvis. Pull your left hip back and right hip forward, bringing your pelvis into a flat plane.

- Inhale. Lift your arms up and out of the shoulders. Stretch long through your fingertips, feeling the energy stretch from one hand to the other.

- Exhale. Lengthen your body over the right leg and fold sideways from the waist. As you fold into Triangle, move the fingers of your right hand onto your leg.

- Breathe and stretch toward the ceiling with the fingers of your left hand. Feel the left side of your body stretch.

- As you develop flexibility, you will continue to slide your right hand down your right leg, eventually grabbing your big toe with your middle and index fingers. This gradual process may take years to achieve. Do not push yourself and distort the integrity of the pose. A pose held at an earlier stage with accuracy and integrity of the posture is yoga, while an extreme pose without integrity is just flexibility.
- Breathe comfortably and deeply. Hold for five to ten deep breaths.
- To exit the pose, inhale and lift through the fingertips of your left hand. Feel your body lift. Then exhale and release your arms. Breathe gently to calm your system.
- Repeat on the opposite side.

(6) Eagle

Eagle is a balance pose that is wonderful for building focus, internal quiet, and a sense of control over the body. It builds poise and nerve coordination. It is also great exercise for the legs and very healing. Yoga theory says that Eagle Pose is great for improving circulation to the legs, thus preventing problems such as spider veins and varicose veins. Two minutes per day of Eagle Pose can work wonders for the strength and flexibility of your legs. It also helps open up the shoulders, chest, and backs of the arms. To perform Eagle Pose:

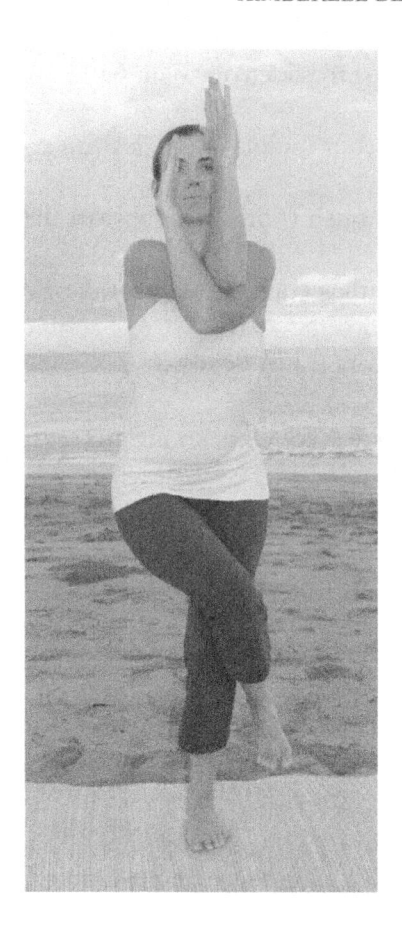

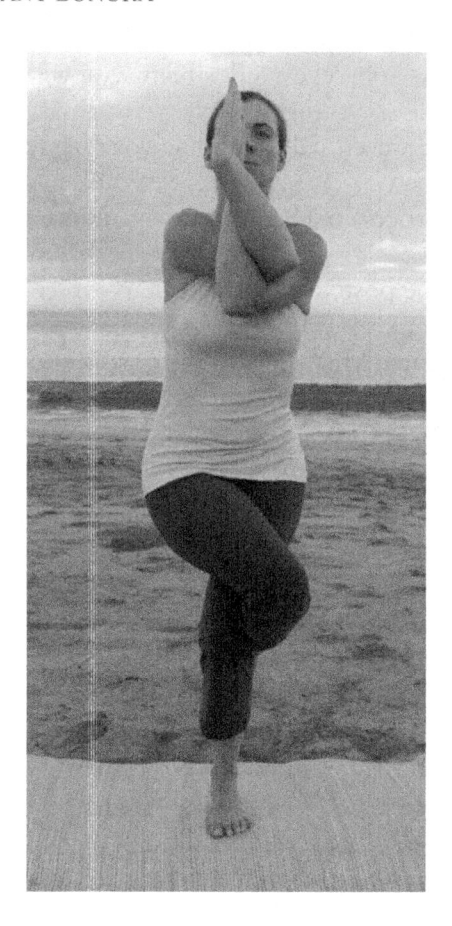

- Start in Mountain Pose. Lift your toes gently to balance the weight over the balls and arches of your feet. Release your toes without putting weight on them and without gripping the mat.

- Shift your balance gently to center your weight on your left leg.

- Cross your right leg over your left. If you can, wrap the right toe behind the left calf, winding your legs up like a pretzel.

- Stretch your right arm in front of you. Then stretch your left arm in front of you, crossing at your elbow over your right arm. Palms should be facing up.

- Keep your elbows connected and lift your arms, bending at the elbows so that your palms face you.

- Rotate your wrists outward so that the tops of the hands face each other. Try to bring the right palm around and under so that you can bring the palms to touch.

- Stay in this pose, breathing and balancing. Hold for five to ten deep breaths.

- Exhale and unwind. Shake out any tension.

- Repeat on the opposite side.

(7) Partial Pigeon

The chest is puffed forward in Pigeon, like a proud pigeon on a stoop. This can be difficult to achieve in the beginning, but suppleness will come with practice. This is a good pose for the hip flexors and hip rotators. If you have a difficult time with the hip flexibility and find your hips hanging in the air, place a rolled blanket or towel under your groin so you have space to rest. To perform Partial Pigeon:

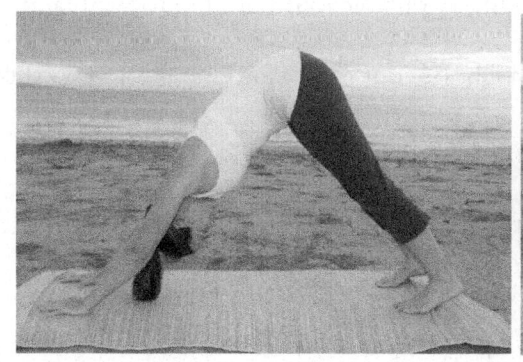

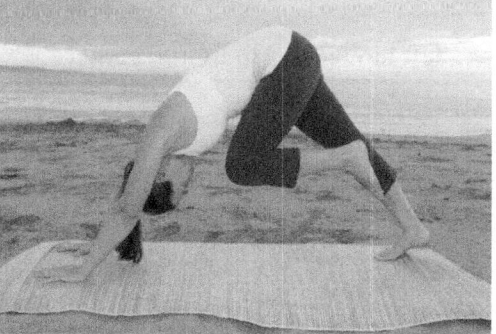

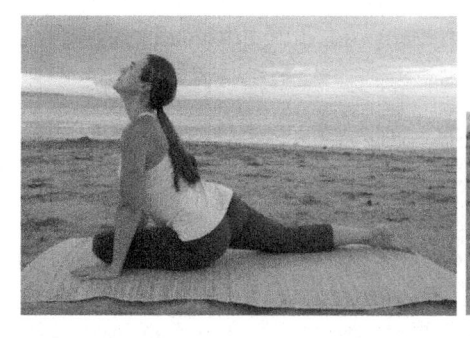

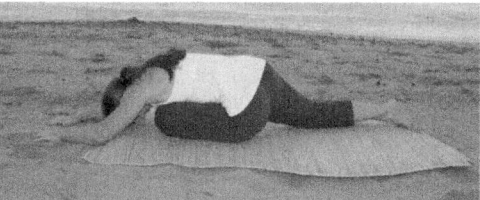

- Start in Downward Dog: on your hands and knees, hands under shoulders, knees under hips, middle fingers stretched forward, palms pressed firmly into the ground. Inhale, lift your hips, and straighten your knees while you stretch the legs back. Keeping the hands grounded, push your weight back toward your heels. Feel your spine lengthen.

- While in Downward Dog, inhale and lift your left foot off the ground. Bring your knee into your chest and hover in that pose.

- Breathe gently, strengthening the abdominals. Then inhale and bring your knee forward, placing it between your hands and resting your shin on the mat.

- Sit in this pose. Work to square your hips by pulling your right hip forward and your left hip back. Attempt to center the weight of your groin onto the floor. You should feel a good stretch on the outside of your left buttocks and upper leg.

- Place your hands on each side of your left knee. Firmly press your hands into the ground as you lift your chest and roll your shoulders back. Feel the sense of openness in your chest and spine. Breathe deeply for five deep breaths.

- Exhale and slide your arms out. Rest your head on the ground if possible; otherwise rest it on knee. This pose is called Nesting Pigeon. Try to find a sense of comfort and stability in the pose. Rest if you can. Hold for five deep breaths.

- Inhale and ground the hands on each side of your chest again. Lift your chest and lengthen the spine.

- Remaining strong through your arms, push through your palms to lift your upper body so that you can lift your left knee off the ground. Then return your left foot to the ground in Downward Dog.

- Breathe in Downward Dog for five deep breaths.

- Repeat on the right side.

(8) Sleeping Big-Toe Cycle

Sleeping Big-Toe Cycle is a great leg stretch. It opens the groin and stretches the legs. It can also release problems with lower back issues and sciatica. Do not get discouraged if this one is hard; do what you can in this pose, as in all poses. Sleeping Big-Toe Cycle is a modified version of a classical Ashtanga pose. To perform it:

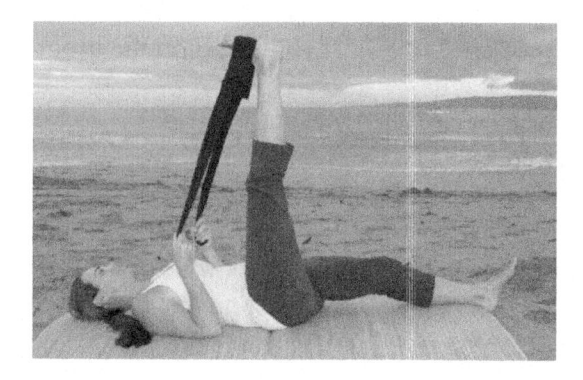

- Lie flat on your back. Put a yoga strap (or a long necktie or ribbon) around your right foot, holding the ends of the strap evenly in both hands.

- Inhale and lift your right foot toward the ceiling. Keep your shoulders grounded and even on the floor. Try not to lift one side. Keep your left leg straight and grounded on the floor with your knee straight.

- Use the strap to pull your right foot toward your face, stretching your leg. Keep both legs straight.

- Breathe deeply for five to ten deep breaths, holding the pose. Relax deeper into the pose, and let your leg gently sink toward your face.

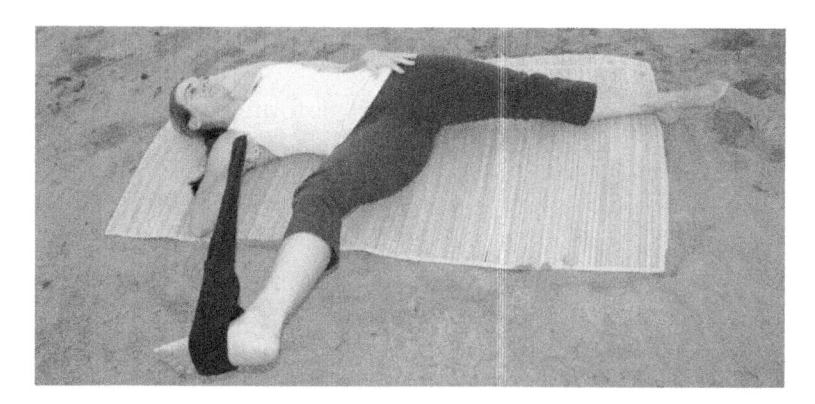

- Take the strap in your right hand. On your next exhalation, open your right leg out to the right. Hold your leg as straight as possible, extending to waist-level. Take your left hand to your left hip and ground your hip down, so that your pelvis is even and in line.

- Look over your left shoulder, away from the open foot, to deepen the stretch. Breathe deeply for five to ten deep breaths.

- Inhale and lift the leg to center. Pull it toward your face again. Breathe deeply. Hold for five to ten deep breaths.

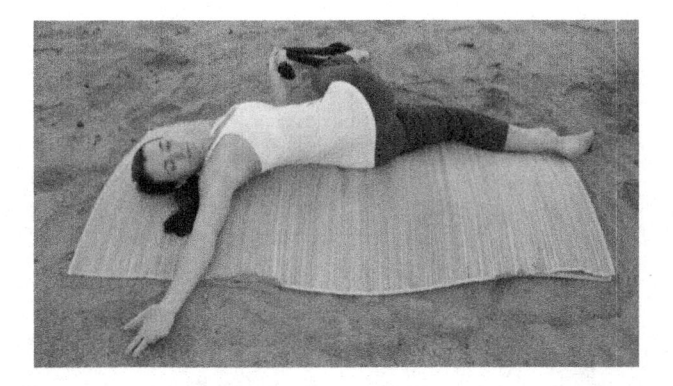

- Take the strap in your left hand. Exhale and cross your right leg to the left side of your body. This movement stretches the outside of your buttocks and leg. Breathe and hold this pose for five to ten deep breaths. (Your hips will move off center in this position, which is normal.)

- Inhale and lift your leg to center.

- Exhale. Release your foot and relax.

- Repeat on the opposite side.

Supportive Exercise for the Back

(1) Standing Spinal Rolls

This pose is an excellent spinal and total body warm-up. It is a great way to start the morning because it energizes your entire being, charging you from head to toe with life and a sense of calm well-being. The more flexible your spine is, the younger your body will look and feel. The undulating motion puts you in touch with the quiet flow of spirit, opening your heart and body to the day. To perform Standing Spinal Rolls:

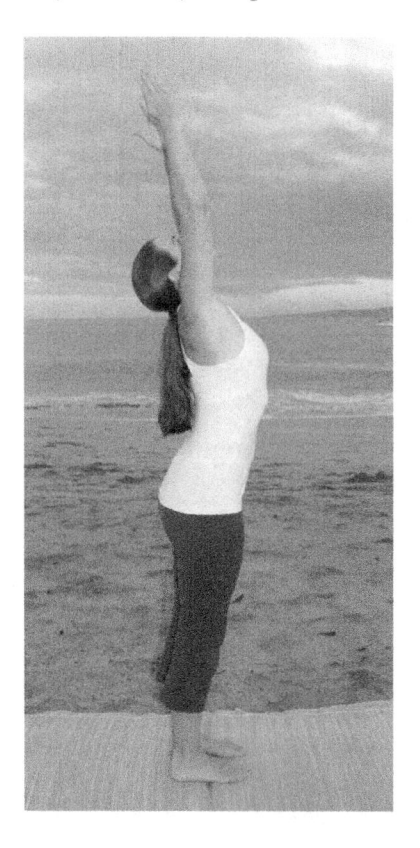

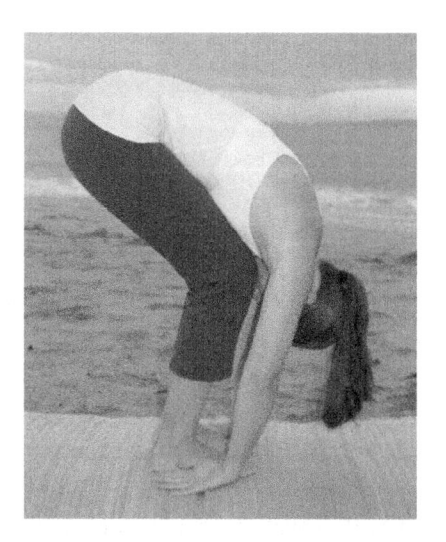

- Begin in Mountain Pose, standing with your toes together and heels apart. Tuck your tailbone under and belly in for a long, lean line of your torso. Tuck in your chin slightly and stretch the back of your neck. Breathe.

- Inhale. Lift your arms over your head, stretching through your fingertips. Keep your shoulders away from your ears as you lift your chest and look up.

- Bend your knees. Exhale and slowly fold your body forward, relaxing your chest on your thighs.

- Release all your weight, gently hanging down with your arms loose, your chest still resting on your thighs, and your head and neck relaxed. Breathe.

- Inhale. With your knees still bent, begin to roll up through the spine—one vertebra at a time. Stack the spine on top of itself, rolling your shoulders and head up last.

- Exhale and pause.

- Inhale and lift again, continuing the cycle. Repeat for two minutes—inhale lifting, exhale folding, inhaling rolling up, and exhale pausing.

(2) Cow-Face Pose

Cow-Face Pose is a great shoulder stretch. It lengthens the arm and opens up the whole of the back. It also encourages diaphragmatic breathing. When you do it, one side will always be more flexible than the other—remember that, so you do not get frustrated when one side does not seem to move. Be patient with your body in this pose. Above all things, yoga teaches patience. To do this exercise:

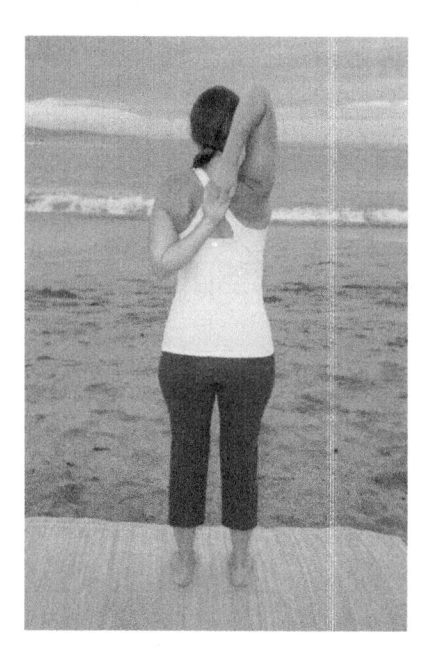

- Stand in a comfortable position with legs hip-width apart.

- Inhale. Lift your right arm straight out of the shoulder.

- Exhale and fold your hand down the center of your upper back. Flatten your palm against your back between your shoulder blades. Pull back through your elbow, so that your arm and elbow do not put pressure on your neck.

- To stretch your shoulder in preparation for Cow-Face, move your left hand to the right elbow, and gently press your right hand farther down your back. Hold and breathe.

- Inhale; stretch your left arm out to the side.

- Bend your left arm at the elbow and fold it up the center of the back with your palm facing up.

- Stretch your right hand down your back and your left hand up the center of the back, moving your fingers toward each other until they eventually touch. Your goal is touching fingers, and eventually, clasping hands.

- Breathe deeply. Hold for five to ten deep breaths.

- Exhale and release.

- Repeat on the opposite side.

(3) Seated Spinal Twist

Twists are wonderful for stretching the lower back. They help with sciatica issues because they release tension in the buttocks and upper thighs where tightness can aggravate the sciatic nerve. Twists also stimulate the digestive system, improving nutritional processing and preventing problems with constipation or diarrhea. Regular practice of twists brings fresh blood to the internal organs, improving overall health of the liver, spleen, kidneys, and lungs. With the leg crossing over, you anchor your pelvis to facilitate a complete side stretch. To do this pose:

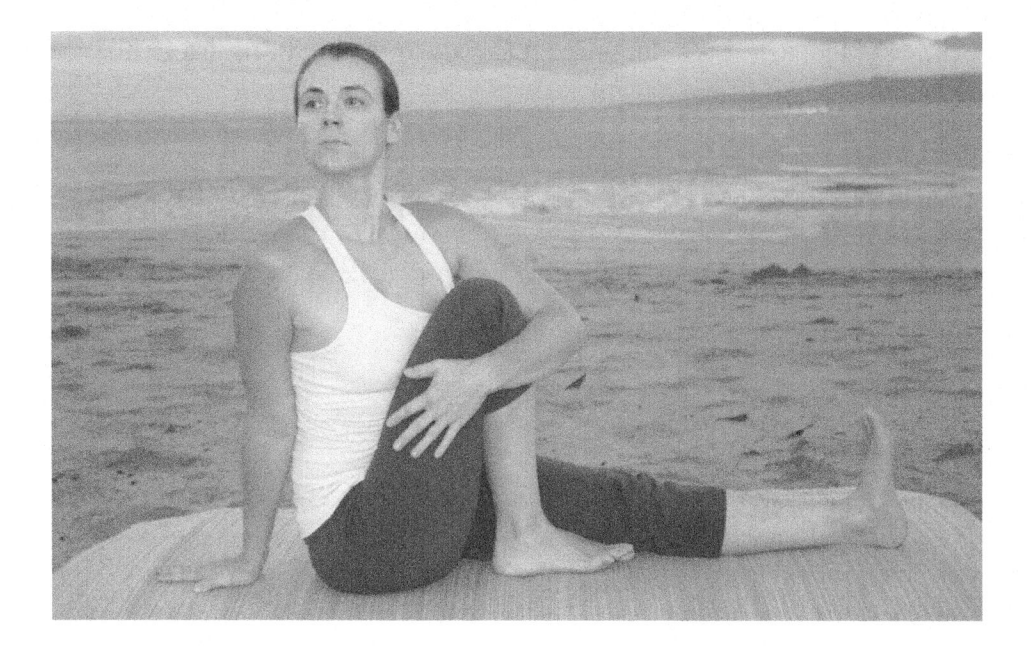

- Sit on the floor. Stretch your legs long and straight. Pull your toes toward the face. Lift your back and keep a straight spine. Open and lift your chest

- Bend your right leg at the knee, planting your right foot solidly on the floor beside your left knee.

- Bring your left hand to the outside of your right knee. Take your right hand behind you. Gently twist, using your left hand to rotate your body. The twist originates from your waist. Rotate your head last. Do not automatically look over your right shoulder; let your exhales take you deeper into the twist until your head gently moves into the position of looking over the shoulder.

- Breathe deeply, moving deeper into the pose with each exhalation, for five to ten deep poses.

- Relax and release to center. Breathe deeply.

- Repeat on the opposite side.

(4) Cobra

Cobra relieves backache problems, invigorates the sympathetic nervous system, normalizes adrenal function, and alleviates constipation. When done with proper form, it also strengthens the upper and mid-back and stretches the chest to open the lungs and improve posture. To complete the Cobra:

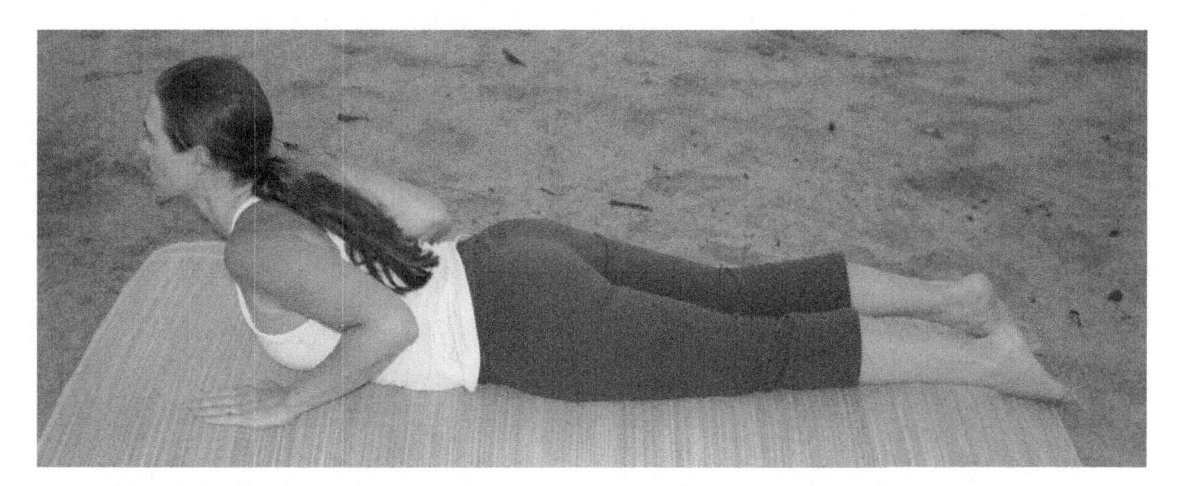

- Begin by lying on your belly.
- Bring your hands to each side of your chest. Plant your palms flatly and solidly into the ground.
- Keep your lower body relaxed but strong. Pull your legs together with your toes touching.
- Inhale; lift your chest and upper chest, using the strength of your back. When you first begin, only lift as far as you can with the strength of your back. Hover your

hands, but do not put weight on them. Feel your chest and chin lifting. Stretch your throat.

- Exhale, release to the mat, and relax.

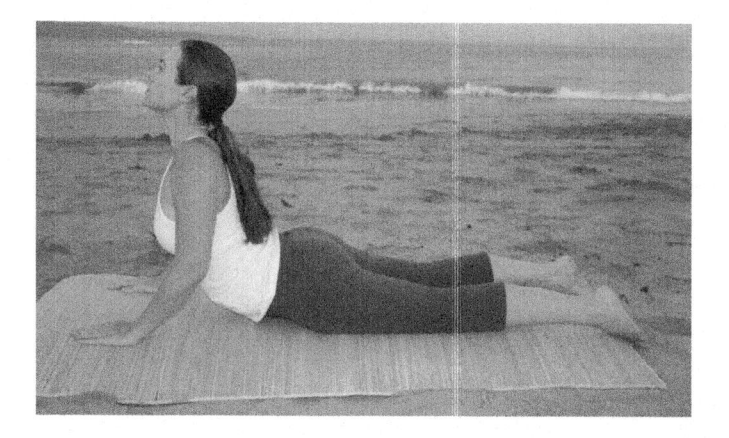

- Moving farther into the pose, inhale and lift. This time press your hands gently into the mat to deepen the stretch. Begin to lift the chest off the mat, slowly straightening your arms if you can. Make sure you keep your hips firmly grounded on the floor.

- When you are in Cobra, it is important to roll your shoulders back and away from your ears, while pulling your chest forward and chin up. Pull your shoulder blades toward one another, down the center of the back. This strengthens your mid-back and helps open your chest.

(5) Bow

Bow massages the abdominal organs, improves digestion, and strengthens thighs, buttocks, and back. Bow also opens the chest, thus improving posture, and stimulates the thyroid gland, thus boosting the metabolism and facilitating healthy weight. To perform Bow:

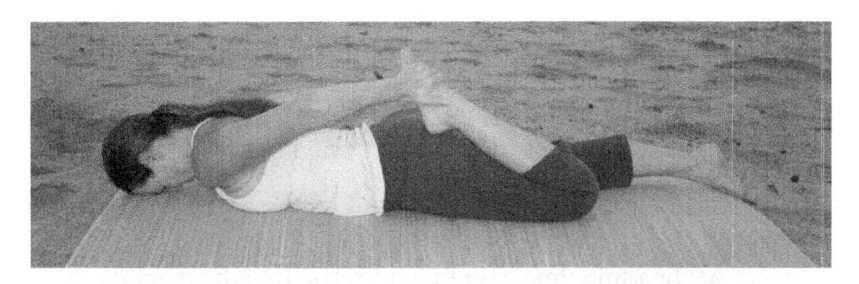

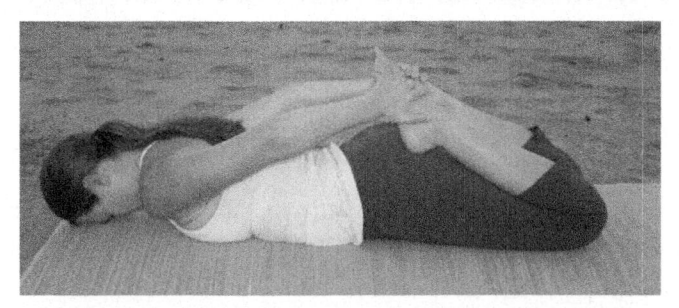

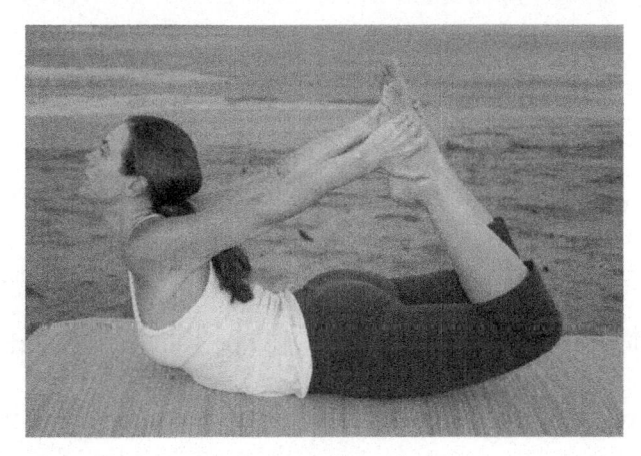

- Start by lying on your stomach.

- Rest your chin gently on the mat. Relax your upper body.

- Lift your left leg behind you, taking the top of your foot in the left hand. Pull your left foot into your bottom. Stretch while keeping the right side of your body relaxed.

- Release your left foot and relax.

- Stretch your right side, taking the foot in your right hand and pulling your heel toward your body. Keep your left side relaxed.

- Release your right foot and relax.

- Lift both feet, taking tops of your feet in your hands, and pulling your heels into your bottom. At the same time, continue to relax. Breathe. Feel the fronts of your thighs stretching. Breathe deeply.

- Inhale and lift through your arms and legs, pulling your body to rest on your belly.

- Try to stay in Bow for five to ten deep breaths. Feel yourself lift a little more and stretch a little deeper with each breath.

- Exhale, release, and relax.

(6) Chinese Ancestor Worship

Chinese Ancestor Worship is an important pose to practice after intense backbends such as Cobra and Bow. It stretches the back in the opposite direction, therefore giving the counter-stretch and releasing residual tension. Chinese Ancestor Worship also stretches the tops of the feet. For healthier feet and better overall health, stretch your feet in poses like Chinese Ancestor Worship. To perform this exercise:

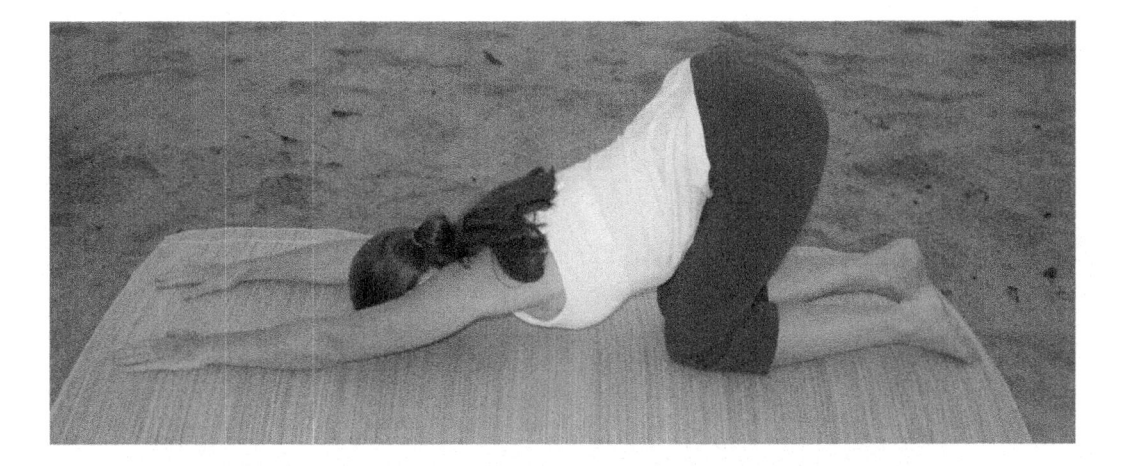

- From lying on your belly, keep the tops of your feet and your shins flat onto the ground.

- Inhale and push off with your hands as you lift your hips and move your upper body back toward your thighs. At the same time, keep your hips lifted. Stretch your arms with your fingers reaching away from you. Bring your forehead to rest on the floor. Feel the sides of your body stretching and lengthening from fingertip to waist.

- Breathe. Feel the stretch and relax into the pose for five to ten deep breaths.

- Relax and release.

(7) Reclining Twist (Knees Bent)

The Reclining Twist is a relaxing pose. It is good for releasing tension and feeling the lower back open up and release. This also trims the waistline and tones the inner thighs. Reclining twist is a nice, gentle twist for postnatal women, to help reestablish your pre-pregnancy figure. To do this pose:

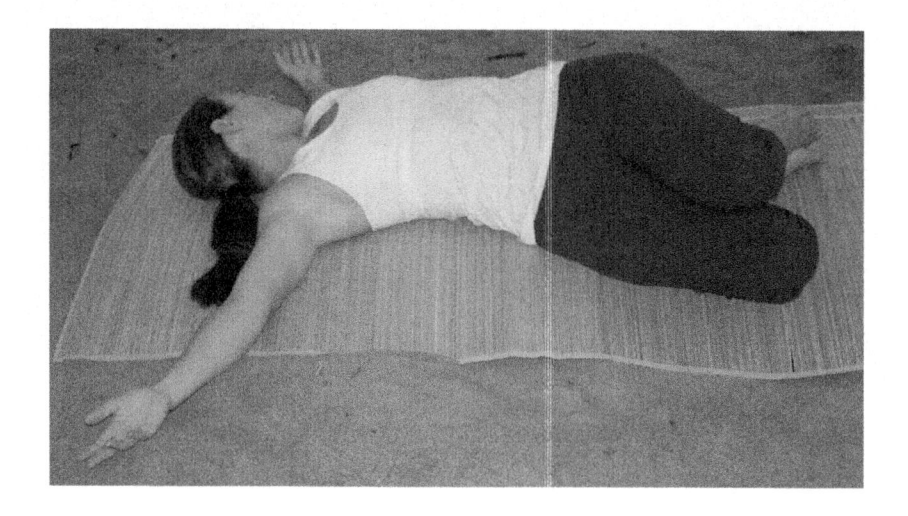

- Lie flat on your back.

- Inhale, lift your knees, and hug them into your chest.

- Hold your knees into your chest and wrap your arms around them. Then gently rock back and forth from side to side, giving yourself a gentle back massage.

- Roll your knees over to the right side of your body, bringing your knees to rest on the side of your body. Stack your left knee on top of the right.

- Stretch your arms from the shoulders, trying to keep your shoulders grounded into the floor.

- Look over your left fingertips, feeling the gentle twist in your body.

- Breathe deeply, holding the pose for five to ten deep breaths.

- With a gentle lift as you inhale, bring your knees to center, hugging them into your chest again. Hold and rest.

- Exhale, roll your knees over to your left side, and repeat.

(8) Supported Backbend

Supported poses are part of a practice called Restorative Yoga. In supportive yoga poses, props, such as bolsters, yoga balls, or blankets, are used to support the body in a gentle version of the pose. This allows you to hold a pose much longer than you would be able to hold the pose on your own. Even though the pose is very simple, because you hold it for a long period of time—up to five, ten, or even fifteen minutes—it can bring deep, healing benefits. In a supported back bend, the chest reaches a deep level of opening, improving posture and encouraging emotional healing. To perform a Supported Backbend:

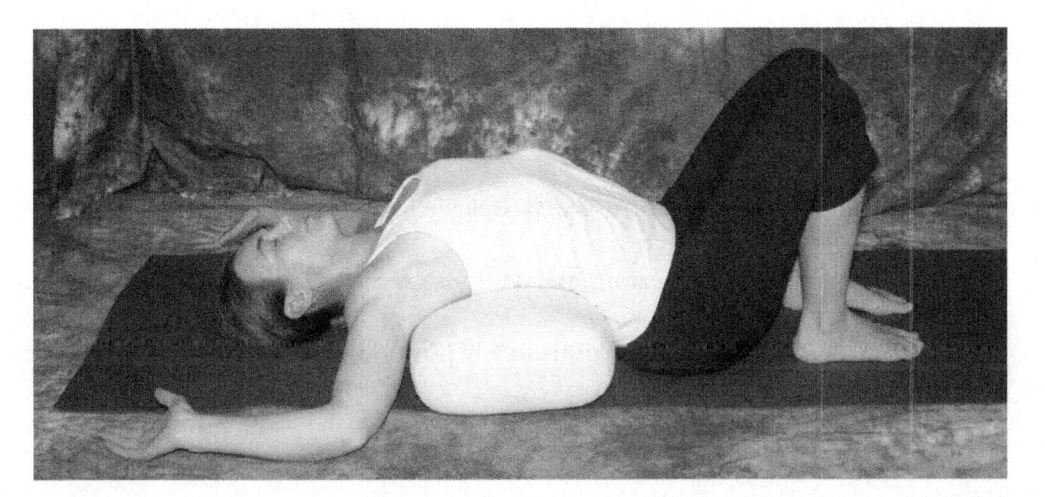

- Find something with a comfortable height for your level of back flexibility. If your back is stiff, fold one or two blankets into a soft cylinder. For more flexibility, use a large, firm pillow or a yoga bolster. For even more flexibility, use a yoga ball.

- Sit against the bottom of the blankets, bolsters, or ball.

- Fold your body back and over the support system, so that you come into a gentle back bend with support for the length of your spine. Your shoulders, neck, and head will gently spill over the top of your supportive prop.

- Relax into the pose and find a sense of comfort. Breathe deeply, in and out, holding the pose for up to fifteen minutes.

- When you finish the pose, your body will be tired from intense effort. Relax and release gently. Rest quietly on your back for several minutes to allow your back muscles to relax and calm down after such intense exercise.

Yoga Walking Pelvic Floor Exercise

Yoga Walking Pelvic Floor Exercise challenges your pelvic strength more than any other pose. The ability to walk and perform pelvic floor contractions must be cultivated. Be patient with yourself and do not get frustrated. Believe in your ability to reach this goal and keep trying. As you learn how to perform pelvic floor exercise while walking, you will find yourself to perform pelvic floor contractions in any position, doing anything else, whenever and wherever you are. This is when you have achieved true pelvic strength. To do this exercise:

- Begin in Mountain Pose. Stand with your feet together, toes touching, heels slightly apart, and body weight centered over your arches.

- Roll your shoulders back and release your arms comfortably to the sides of your body.
- Activate the muscles of your upper thighs by lifting them into your hips to strengthen and tone, as well as protect your knees.
- Your spine should be long and fluid. Make your neck long and relaxed with your chin tucked in slightly to open the back of your neck.
- Tuck your tailbone and torso into the core of your body. Feel your body strong and balanced and your spine straight and long. Ground your feet firmly into the earth.
- While maintaining correct posture and spinal alignment, begin walking at a calm, steady pace.
- At this point, become aware of your pelvic muscles. Begin pelvic floor contractions and contract your pelvic muscles up.
- Hold for five seconds.
- Release and relax five seconds.
- Repeat two more times (for three five-second Contract, five-second Releases in a row).
- Rest thirty seconds.
- Repeat another cycle.

- Build this one-minute cycle up to fifteen minutes of Yoga Walking. (You will work up to fifteen minutes of walking, with three Contract-Releases per minute, for a total of forty-five Contract Releases in one session).

Pelvic Floor Meditation

The pelvic floor tends to hold residual tension on a regular basis. This residual tension prevents you from relaxing the pelvic muscles, which makes them more prone to fatigue. When your pelvic muscles are fatigued, you are more likely to experience problems with incontinence. When pelvic muscles are "too tired," it becomes difficult to hold the urethral sphincter closed, and urine can leak. Therefore, it is very important to practice pelvic relaxation, learning to release completely the pelvic floor.

Whenever you exercise or perform strengthening exercises, your body needs an equal amount of relaxation. According to Kundalini Yoga theory, it is during this rest that your body experiences the results of your practice. It is also during this rest that your body heals. Without the rest portion, pelvic floor exercise is ineffective. Relaxation can be the most important part of any yoga practice. The final relaxation allows your body to absorb the energy released by the asanas and gain the full benefits of yoga practice.

When you first begin the practice of Pelvic Floor Meditation, start with Spread Legs up the Wall Pose, even if you are more advanced. Learn the feel of a relaxed pelvic floor.

(1) Beginner: Spread Legs up the Wall Pose

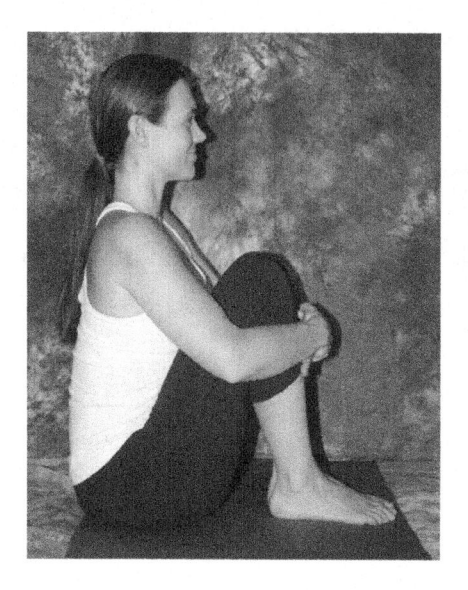

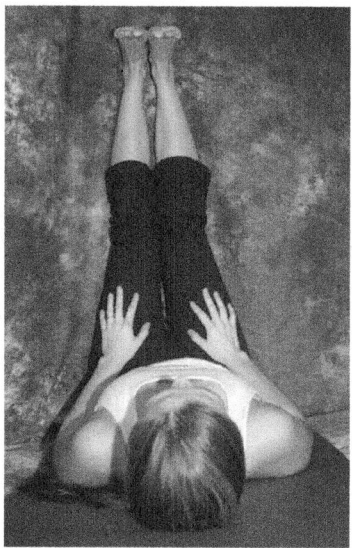

- Sit sideways against a wall with the sides of one hip and shoulder/arm against the wall.

- Carefully, turn your body so that your legs prop against the wall. Recline onto your back.

- If you have moved away from the wall, use the strength of your hands and arms to gently lift your body and slide your hips closer to the wall.

- You should feel comfortable in this position. If necessary, place a cushion or a blanket under your lower back or tailbone for support. You may want a pillow under your head or neck as well.

- Rest completely.

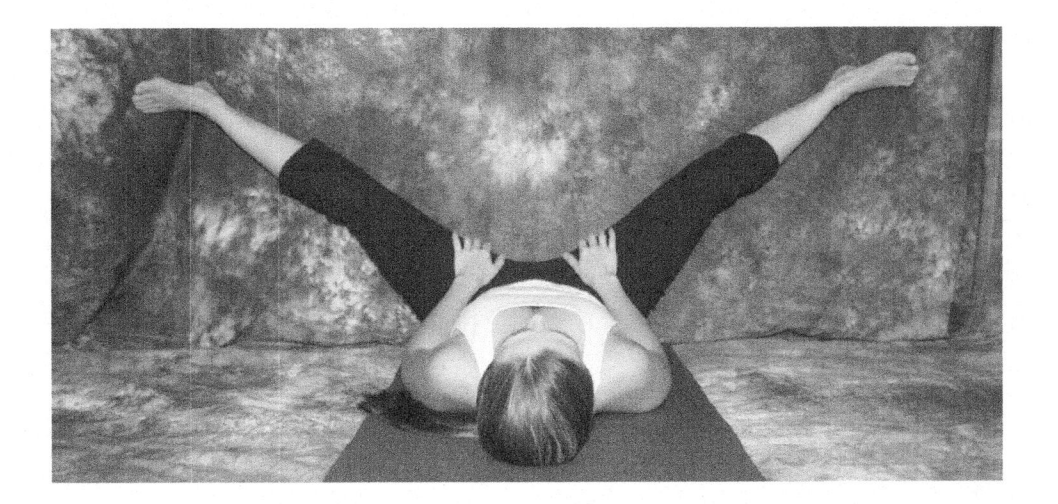

- Spread your legs gently. If you are not used to Spread Legs up the Wall Pose, you may find your inner thighs stretching beyond your capacity and causing cramps in your buttocks or outer thighs. To prevent this, you can use a yoga strap (or a cotton belt or necktie). Tie the strap around your ankles, leaving enough slack for a comfortable, complete stretch of your inner thighs and groin. Make sure it is sufficiently tight enough to support your legs against one another and prevent the strain caused by over stretching. Alternatively, you can tie the strap around your lower thighs, just above your knee. Try both positions and use whichever is more comfortable for you.

- Place your hands in the groin area, feeling your pelvic muscles. Learn to feel this area while you are completely relaxed—no tension, no pressure, and no contraction whatsoever.

- Focus your concentration on the pelvic region of your body, feeling the energy of your hands healing and soothing your pelvic floor.

- Breathe rhythmically and calmly, clearing your mind and body of tension.

- Hold for fifteen minutes, if possible, releasing the pose if it becomes uncomfortable.

- To release Spread Legs up the Wall Pose, place the palms of your hands on the outside of your thighs.

- Using the strength of your hands and arms, push your legs together. Perform a pelvic floor contraction at Level Two to reestablish pelvic control and prevent urinary leakage.

- Rest with both legs up the wall and your thighs together.

- When you are ready, bend your knees and bring your thighs to your chest, wrapping your arms around the outside of your knees. Rest.

- Perform a pelvic floor exercise at Level Two to reestablish pelvic control and prevent urinary leakage. Hold the pelvic floor exercise for urinary control. Then roll onto your right side, resting completely on the side of your body, letting your back, legs, and pelvis melt into the floor.

- Finally, place your palms against the ground. Using the strength of your arms, rather than your back, push yourself to a seated position.

- Take a moment to reflect on your Pelvic Yoga practice. Reap the rewards of your committed effort. Focus your awareness on the effort you are making to improve your life and health. Feel positive about that effort, productive about the time spent in Pelvic Yoga practice, and happy about the results you are already achieving.

- Release. Namaste.

(2) Moderate & Advanced: Reclined Cobbler's Pose

When you are comfortable with Pelvic Floor Meditation in Spread Legs up the Wall pose, you can try to achieve relaxation in Reclined Cobbler's Pose. Reclined Cobbler's Pose is an excellent posture for pelvic issues of any kind. Women experiencing menstrual cramps or difficulties will find Reclined Cobbler's Pose beneficial for pain relief and soothing comfort. Whether sitting or reclined, Cobbler's Pose increases blood flow and relaxation to the entire pelvic region. To do this:

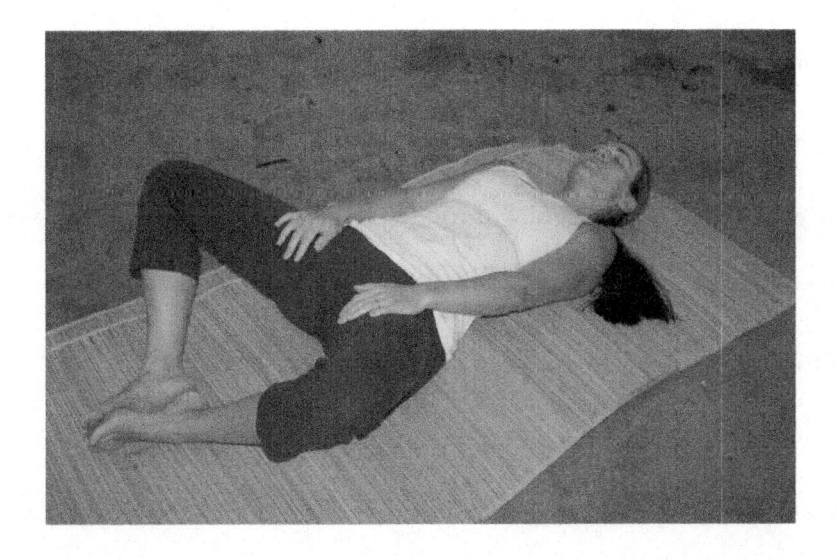

- Sitting on the floor with a straight back, bring the soles of your feet together and pull your heels toward your thighs.

- Breathing deeply, hold your toes. Maintaining a straight back, feel the outward rotation of your thigh muscles. Concentrate on opening your groin.

- Then, gently relax back onto your elbows. Keeping your feet together and pulled in toward your groin, slowly release onto your back. Relax your arms out to your sides and rest your back fully on the ground. Concentrate to feel the full length of your spine.

- If your legs and hips experience discomfort, place a blanket or a pillow underneath each knee for support. Be sure to keep your thighs open but use enough support to prevent muscle strain.

- Rest your hands gently on the insides of your thighs, right at your pelvis. Feel with your fingers the line where the leg connects to the hip.

- Completely relax your groin and pelvic area.

- Close your eyes and relax, going through the Pelvic Floor Meditation as practiced in the beginner-level relaxation pose.

- Rest for ten to fifteen minutes.

- When you come out of Reclined Cobbler's pose, your legs and pelvic floor muscles will be very tired. Perform a pelvic floor exercise at Level Two and hold to prevent any possible leakage.

- Use your hands to lift each knee to center.

- Remain lying on your back with your knees bent and feet flat on the ground. Rest your thighs.

- Perform a pelvic floor exercise at Level Two and hold to prevent any possible leakage. When you are ready, roll onto your right side. Relax into the floor, completely resting your body.

- Finally, place your palms against the ground. Using the strength of your arms, rather than your back, push yourself to a seated position.

- Take a moment to reflect on your Pelvic Yoga practice. Focus your awareness on the effort you are making to improve your life and health. Feel positive about your work, productive about the time spent in Pelvic Yoga practice, and happy about the results you are already feeling.

- Release. Namaste.

Pelvic Yoga Quick Guide: Using Yoga for Pelvic Health
Kimberlee Bethany Bonura, PhD, RYT

The information provided is intended as helpful information for preventative bladder and pelvic health. It is not intended to diagnose or treat any medical condition. Medical conditions should be discussed with a doctor, preferably an urogynecologist or an urologist specializing in rehabilitation. Before beginning this or any exercise program, consult your doctor. Pregnant women and those with chronic injuries should never begin an exercise program without the permission of their physician.

Pelvic Floor Exercise: A contraction of the pelvic floor muscles to build strength and tone the entire pelvic region. Find your perineum—the space between the anus and the genitals. Contract, pulling it into your body cavity, as if suppressing gas and/or urine.

Pelvic Yoga: Integrating pelvic floor exercise with specific yoga postures for optimum pelvic results.
Benefits: It prevents urinary incontinence, improves and enhances sexuality, and strengthens the entire pelvic region. It is great for pre/postnatal and pre/postmenopausal women.

Three ways to recognize your pelvic floor muscles:
(1) Perform a Stop Test while urinating—not for regular practice!
(2) Do a Finger Test in vagina or rectum.
(3) Ask your gynecologist at your next exam.
Best postures for finding the muscles: Lie on your back with your hands resting over your pubic bone; feel the muscles lift. Alternatively, lying on your side, curl your knees into your chest.

Four Advanced Techniques
(1) Contract-Release—Contract. Hold five seconds. Release five seconds.
(2) Quick-Flick—one to two second pulses
(3) Long Hold—ten-second hold with ten-second rests in between
(4) Elevator—Four floors—Go up, floor-by-floor, holding at each level. Go down, floor by floor, holding at each level. Release to basement for complete relaxation.
Stay calm and relaxed. Remember to breathe. Do not tense your abs, buttocks, or thighs; keep them soft and relaxed.

Goal: Ninety repetitions per day, mixing the four kinds, in various postures.

Pelvic Yoga Postures:
Simple Sitting Contract-Release
Child's Pose Quick-Flicks
Squatting Elevator
Mountain Pose Balance with Long Holds
Yogic Bicycle
Stomach Contractions

Pelvic Floor Meditation:
Legs up the Wall for Relaxation

References

Sandra Anderson and Rolf Sovik, PsyD. *Yoga: Mastering the Basics* (Honesdale, Pennsylvania: The Himalayan Institute Press, 2000), 209.

James F. Balch, MD, and Phyllis A. Balch, *Prescription for Nutritional Healing, 2nd Edition* (Garden City Park, New York: Avery Publishing Group, 1997), 385.

Baron Baptiste, *Journey Into Power: How to Sculpt Your Ideal Body, Free Your True Self, and Transform Your Life With Yoga* (New York: Fireside, 2002), 201.

Kathryn Burgio, K. Lynette Pearce, and Angelo Lucco, *Staying Dry: A Practical Guide to Bladder Control* (Baltimore: Johns Hopkins University Press, 1989), 6–7.

Cherie Calbom and Maureen Keane, *Juicing for Life: A Guide to the Health Benefits of Fresh Fruit and Vegetable Juicing* (Garden City Park, New York: Avery Publishing Group, Inc., 1992), 69.

Thomas Cleary (Translator), *Dhammapada: The Sayings of the Buddha* (New York: Bantam Books, 1995).

Kenneth S. Cohen, *The Way of Qigong: The Art and Science of Chinese Energy Healing* (New York: Ballantine Books, 1997).

Alain Daniélou (Translator), *The Complete Kāma Sūtra: The First Unabridged Modern Translation of the Classic Indian Text* (Rochester, Vermont: Park Street Press, 1994), 97.

Indra Devi, *Renew Your Life Through Yoga* (New York: Warner, 1963), 213.

Harvey and Marilyn Diamond, *Fit for Life* (New York: MJF Books, 1985), 26 – 28.

Adelle Davis, *Let's Get Well* (New York: Signet, 1972/1965), 65.

Arlene Eisenberg, Heidi E. Murkoff, and Sandee E. Hathaway. *What to Expect When You're Expecting* (New York: Workman Publishing, 1991/1984).

Rita Elkins, MH, *Natural Treatments for Urinary Incontinence* (Pleasant Grove, Utah: Woodland Publishing, 2000), 6.

Alice Feinstein (Editor), *Symptoms: Their Causes and Cures: How to Understand and Treat 265 Health Concerns* (Emmaus, Pennsylvania: Rodale Press, 1994), 270.

Mohandas K. Gandhi, *Gandhi's Health Guide* (Freedom, California: The Crossing Press, 2000), 175.

Bill Gottlieb (Editor*), New Choices in Natural Healing: Over 1,800 of the Best Self-Help Remedies from the World of Alternative Medicine* (Emmaus, Pennsylvania: Rodale Press, Inc. 1995).

Alma E. Guinness (Editor), *Reader's Digest Great Health Hints and Handy Tips* (Pleasantville, New York: Reader's Digest Association, Inc., 1994), 370.

Kundalini Yoga with Gurmukh, Living Arts video, 2004.

David Hoffmann, *The New Holistic Herbal: A Herbal Celebrating the Wholeness of Life* (New York: Barnes and Noble Books, 1995/1983), 111.

J. Frank Hurdle, MD, *A Country Doctor's Common Sense Health Manual* (West Nyack, N.Y.: Parker Publishing Company, Inc., 1975).

Incontinence, *Health Digest: Your Total Health Solution*, Winter 2002, 63.

Sandra Jordan, *Yoga for Pregnancy: Safe and Gentle Stretches* (New York: St. Martin's Press, 1987), 7.

Wynn Kapit and Lawrence M. Elson, *The Anatomy Coloring Book, 3rd Edition* (San Francisco: Benjamin Cummings, 2002).

Wynn Kapit, Robert I. Macey, and Esmail Meisami, *The Physiology Coloring Book* (San Francisco: Benjamin/Cummings, 2000).

Diane Kaschak Newman, *The Urinary Incontinence Sourcebook* (Los Angeles: Lowell House, 1999/1997), 287.

Diane Kaschak Newman and Alan J. Wein, *Managing and Treating Urinary Incontinence*, Second Edition. (Health Professions, 2008).

Donald W. Kemper, *Healthwise Handbook: A Self-Care Manual for You, 12th Edition* (Boise, Idaho: Healthwise, Incorporated, 1995).

Shakti Parwha Kaur Khalsa, *Kundalini Yoga: The Flow of Eternal Power* (New York: Perigee, 1996), 95.

Gayla J. Kirschmann and John D. Kirschmann, *Nutrition Almanac, 4th Edition* (New York: McGraw-Hill, 1996 / 1973), 176.

Mark S. Lachs, MD, Caring for Mom and Dad: Battling the Embarrassment of Incontinence, *Prevention Magazine*, August 1998, 173–180.

Jyothi Larson and Ken Howard, *Yoga Mom, Buddha Baby: The Yoga Workout for New Moms* (New York: Bantam Books, 2002), 29.

Niels H. Lauersen, MD, PhD, and Colette Bouchez, *Getting Pregnant: What Couples Need to Know Right Now* (New York: Fawcett Columbine, 1991), 156.

Niels Lauersen, MD, and Steven Whitney, *It's Your Body: A Woman's Guide to Gynecology* (New York: Playboy Paperbacks, 1986/1973), 479.

Frederick Leboyer, *Inner Beauty, Inner Light: Yoga for Pregnant Women* (New York: Newmarket Press, 1997/1978), 182.

Martha Lind, *Yoga at Any Age* (Miami: Martha Lind, Inc., 1971).

Ellen Michaud, Lila L. Anastas, and the Editors of *Prevention* Magazine, *Listen to Your Body: A Head-to-Toe Guide to More than 400 Symptoms, Their Causes, and Best Treatments* (New York: MJF Books, 1988), 435.

Olivia Miller, *The Yoga Deck: Poses and Meditation for Body, Mind, and Spirit*, San Francisco: Chronicle Books, 2001.

National Association for Continence, *Take Control: Incontinence Diagnosis, Treatment, and Management*, 2000.

National Kidney and Urologic Diseases Information Clearinghouse, *Urinary Incontinence in Children*, 1997.

National Kidney and Urologic Diseases Information Clearinghouse, *Urinary Incontinence in Men*, 2001.

Gary Null, *The Complete Question and Answer Book of Natural Therapy* (New York: Robert Speller & Sons, 1972), 78.

Paddy O'Brien, *Yoga for Women: Complete Mind and Body Fitness* (London: Thorsons, 1994/1991), 46.

Adelheid Ohlig, *Luna Yoga: Vital Fertility and Sexuality* (Woodstock, NY: Ash Tree Publishing, 1994).

Linda G. Rector-Page, ND, PhD, *Healthy Healing: An Alternative Healing Reference, 9th Edition* (Healthy Healing Publications, 1994 / 1985), 153.

Lee Rodwell and Andrea Kon, *Natural Pregnancy: The Complete Guide to a Gentle, Natural Pregnancy and a Healthy, Happy Baby* (London: Salamander Books Ltd., 1997).

Personal discussion during physical therapy with Kathleen Roth, Licensed Physical Therapist, El Paso, Texas, 2000.

The Simon Foundation, Understanding Good Bowel Health, *The Informer*, p. 1.

The Sivananda Yoga Centre, *The Book of Yoga: The Complete Step-by-Step Guide* (London: Ebury Press, 1983).

The Sivananda Yoga Vedanta Centre, *101 Essential Tips: Yoga* (New York: DK Publishing, Inc., 1995).

Lendon Smith, MD, *Feed Yourself Right* (New York: Dell Trade Paperback, 1983), 296.

Swami Prabhavananda and Christopher Isherwood (Translators), *Bhagavad-Gita* ("Song of God") (New York: Barnes and Noble Books, 1995, originally Hollywood: Vedanta Society of Southern California, 1944), 9.

His Divine Grace A.C. Bhaktivedanta Swami Prabhupāda, *The Perfection of Yoga* (New York: The Bhaktivedanta Book Trust, 1976/1972), 17.

Jess Stearn, *Yoga, Youth, & Reincarnation* (Malibu, CA: Valley of the Sun, 1993/1965).

Carolyn J. Strange, "Incontinence Can Be Controlled," *The US Food and Drug Administration Website* at http://www.fda.gov/fdac/features/1997/597_urin.html

David Swenson. *Ashtanga Yoga: The Practice Manual* (Houston, TX: Ashtanga Yoga Productions, 2000).

Wendy Teasdill, *Yoga for Pregnancy* (Chicago: Contemporary Books 2000).

Louise Tenney, *The Encyclopedia of Natural Remedies* (Pleasant Grove, Utah: Woodland Publishing Inc., 1995), 20.

Louise Tenney, *Health Handbook, 2nd Edition* (Pleasant Grove, Utah: Woodland Books, 1994), 15.

Tranquility, *Dealing with Incontinence: Straight Facts about Bladder Control and Incontinence Products* (Dunbridge, Ohio: Principle Business Enterprises, Inc.), 1.

Elizabeth Vierck, *7 Steps to Normal Bladder Control: Simple, Practical Tips and Techniques for Staying Dry* (Gig Harbor, Washington: Harbor Press, 1998), 29.

Swami Kriyananda (J. Donald Walters), *The Art and Science of Raja Yoga* (Nevada City, California: Crystal Clarity Publishers, 2002), 308–309.

Michael A. Weiner, *Earth Medicine, Earth Food: Plant Remedies, Drugs, and Natural Foods of the North American Indians* (New York: Fawcett Columbine, 1980/1972), 83–84.

Stella Weller, *Complete Yoga: The Gentle and Effective Way to Health and Well-Being* (New York: Barnes & Noble Books, 2001).

Douglas Wile, *Art of the Bedchamber: The Chinese Sexual Yoga Classics, Including Women's Solo Meditation Texts* (Albany, New York: State University of New York Press, 1992), 25.

Merryl Winstein, *Your Fertility Signals: Using Them to Achieve or Avoid Pregnancy, Naturally* (St. Louis, Missouri: Smooth Stone Press, 1997 / 1989).

F. Yeats-Brown, *Yoga Explained* (New York: Vista House, 1958 / 1937).

Paramahansa Yogananda, *Man's Eternal Quest* (Los Angeles: Self-Realization Fellowship, 1992/1975), 152.

Suggested Internet Resources

American Congress of Obstetricians and Gynecologists: http://www.acog.org/~/media/for%20patients/faq081.ashx

Mayo Clinic: http://www.mayoclinic.com/health/urinary-incontinence/DS00404

Medline Plus: http://www.nlm.nih.gov/medlineplus/urinaryincontinence.html

National Association for Continence: http://www.nafc.org/

National Institutes of Health, National Institute on Aging: http://www.nia.nih.gov/health/publication/urinary-incontinence

National Kidney and Urologic Diseases Information Clearinghouse (NKUDIC): http://kidney.niddk.nih.gov/index.aspx

Society of Urologic Nurses and Associates: http://www.suna.org

US Department of Health and Human Services, Office on Women's Health: http://www.womenshealth.gov/publications/our-publications/fact-sheet/urinary-incontinence.cfm

Web MD: http://www.webmd.com/urinary-incontinence-oab/default.htm

Index

Airplane 76
Angle Balance 68, 73
anus 2, 3, 4, 7, 8, 12, 18, 116
Ashtanga yoga 18, 19
Balance 11, 34, 48, 49, 68, 73
Basement 15
Boat Pose 73
Bow 100, 102
Breathwork 16
Bridge Pose 50
bulbospongiosus 2, 4
Camel 39, 40, 41
Cat-Cow 26, 58
cervix 19
Chair 29, 31
chakra 18, 20, 61
Child's Pose 28, 29
Chinese Ancestor Worship 102
Cobbler's Pose 47, 71, 72, 113
Cobra 99, 100, 102
coccyx 5
Contract-Release 10, 12, 24, 26, 38, 39, 40, 41, 42, 71, 116
Corpse Pose 36
Cow-Face Pose 95
Crescent Pose 81
Downward Facing Dog 57
Eagle 87
Elevators 10, 13, 34, 36, 37, 46, 47, 48, 71
external sphincter ani 2, 4
figure eight 4, 5, 6, 53
Finger Test 8
Fish Pose 59
Frog Pose 42
Happy Baby 53, 55, 120

incontinence .. 1, 3, 4, 14, 23, 54, 109, 116, 122
Kegel 3, 18
Kundalini .. 18, 19, 20, 21, 23, 66, 67, 109, 118, 119
level two 14
Locust 77
Long Holds 10, 13, 31, 32, 34, 48, 50, 52
menopause 2, 3
menstruation 23
Mountain Pose 34, 79, 82, 86, 88, 95, 106
Mul Bandh 19, 21, 22, *See* Mulabandha or root lock
Mulabandha 18, 19, 64
Patanjali's Yoga Sutras 16
Pelvic Floor Meditation 109, 113, 116
pelvic hammock 64
pelvic relaxation 109
Pelvic Yoga Bicycle 70
penis 2, 6, 8, 12
Perfect Posture 38
perineum 3, 5, 8, 9, 18, 116
Pigeon 89, 91
prana 18
pregnancy 1, 2, 3, 26, 44, 45, 103
   childbirth 3
prostate 3, 4, 6
pubococcygeus 2
Qigong 4, 117
Quick-Flicks . 10, 12, 14, 28, 29, 31, 42, 43, 44, 45, 63
Reclining Twist 103
rectum .... *See* anus
Restorative Yoga 105
root lock ..... 18, 19, 20, 22, 23, *See* Mulabandha
Sat Kriya 21, 22

123

Seated Spinal Twist 97	Stop Test 7
sexual intercourse 4	Supported Backbend 105
Side-Angle Pose 84	Tree Pose 48
Simple sitting 24	Triangle 85, 86
Sitting Twists 67	Uddyiana Bandha 64
Sleeping Big-toe cycle 91	urethra 2, 3, 4, 5, 6, 7, 12
solar plexus 64	vagina .... v, 2, 3, 4, 5, 8, 116
sphincter 2, 4, 12, 109	Warrior One 78
Spread Legs up the Wall 109, 110, 111, 112, 113	Warrior Two 82
Squatting 44, 45, 47	Wheel 61, 62, 63
Staff Pose 31	Wide-leg Sitting Forward Bend 53
Standing Spinal Rolls 94	Wind-Relieving Pose 32
Stomach Contractions 23, 64	yoga bandhas 18
Stomach lock ...... 23, *See* stomach contractions	Yoga Walking Pelvic Floor Exercise 106

About the Author

Kimberlee Bethany Bonura, PhD, Registered Yoga Teacher, provides a full spectrum of yoga, fitness, and wellness consulting services. Dr. Bonura is available for both individual and organizational/corporate consulting, professional speaking engagements, professional and personal development workshops, and ongoing fitness and wellness coaching.

Kimberlee Bethany Bonura earned her PhD in Educational Psychology from Florida State University, with a research focus in Sport & Exercise Psychology, and graduate certificates in Program Evaluation and Educational Measurement and Statistics. Her doctoral dissertation, The Impact of Yoga on Psychological Health in Older Adults, won national awards from the American Psychological Association (Division 47) and the Association for Applied Sport Psychology.

Dr. Bonura has been practicing yoga for over twenty years and teaching yoga since 1997. She is a triple-certified yoga instructor, registered with the Yoga Alliance, and a member of the International Association of Yoga Therapists. She is also a certified personal trainer (Aerobics and Fitness Association of America), a certified group fitness instructor (International Fitness Professionals Association), a certified group kickboxing instructor (AFAA), a certified tai chi / Qi gong instructor (IFPA), a certified senior fitness specialist (IFPA), a certified weight management instructor (IFPA), certified in prenatal and youth fitness (AFAA), a certified anger resolution therapist (CAR), and a Reiki master in the Usui System.

Dr. Bonura has extensive experience as a yoga, fitness, and wellness instructor. She specializes in developing personally tailored plans to promote an individual's well-being and achievement of wellness goals. Dr. Bonura's combined backgrounds in academic research, yoga/fitness/wellness instruction and consulting, and program evaluation provide a unique perspective that allows her to provide comprehensive wellness promotion and performance enhancement services.

Dr. Bonura has published in local, national, and international magazines and academic journals in the topic areas of yoga, health, wellness, fitness, stress management, and performance enhancement. She is the author and lecturer of *How to Stay Fit as You Age* (2013), from The Great Courses (www.thegreatcourses.com). She is a member of the editorial board of the *International Journal of Yoga Therapy*. Previously, she served as Editor-in-Chief of the Yoga Alliance newsletter *Yoga Matters* from 2002–2004. Dr. Bonura has developed specialized yoga programs in Seated/Chair Yoga for Senior Citizens; Pelvic Yoga for pre/post pregnancy, pre/post menopause, incontinence prevention, and sexual enhancement; Power Yoga for Empowerment, designed to encourage self-esteem in teenagers and young adults; and Partner Yoga for family and marital enhancement. She has consulted with individuals and organizations, including elite athletes, institutes of higher education, non-profit community organizations, and corporations.

Website: www.drkimberleebonura.com
Email: info@drkimberleebonura.com

Made in United States
North Haven, CT
23 March 2022